School Phobia, Panic Attacks
and Anxiety in Children

of related interest

Social Awareness Skills for Children
Márianna Csóti
ISBN 1 84310 003 7

Contentious Issues
Discussion Stories for Young People
Márianna Csóti
ISBN 1 84310 033 9

People Skills for Young Adults
Márianna Csóti
ISBN 1 85302 716 2

Helping Children to Build Self-Esteem
A Photocopiable Activities Book
Deborah Plummer
ISBN 1 85302 927 0

Listening to Young People in School, Youth Work
and Counselling
Nick Luxmoore
ISBN 1 85302 909 2

Asperger's Syndrome
A Guide for Parents and Professionals
Tony Attwood
ISBN 1 85302 577 1

New Perspectives on Bullying
Ken Rigby
ISBN 1 85302 872 X

Stop the Bullying
A Handbook for Schools
Ken Rigby
ISBN 1 85302 070 3

School Phobia, Panic Attacks and Anxiety in Children

Márianna Csóti

Jessica Kingsley Publishers
London and Philadelphia

First published in the United Kingdom in 2003
by Jessica Kingsley Publishers
116 Pentonville Road
London N1 9JB, UK
and
400 Market Street, Suite 400
Philadelphia, PA 19106, USA

www.jkp.com

Library of Congress Cataloging in Publication Data
A CIP catalog record for this book is available from the Library of Congress

British Library Cataloguing in Publication Data
A CIP catalogue record for this book is available from the British Library

ISBN-13: 978 0 84310 091 1
ISBN-10: 1 84310 091 6

Printed and Bound in Great Britain by
Athenaeum Press, Gateshead, Tyne and Wear

Contents

*This book is dedicated to my daughter
and all other children who have had, or currently suffer
from, problems outlined in this book.*

*I should like to thank Chris and Fiona Woods for all their
help in our time of need, it remains much appreciated.*

*I should also like to thank Dr Gill Salmon, Consultant
Child and Adolescent Psychiatrist and Senior Lecturer in
Child and Adolescent Mental Health, for her considerable
and invaluable help in the final stages of writing this book.*

Introduction

No official statistics are available for children suffering from school phobia in the UK. However, according to Anxiety Care (see *Useful Contacts*) the number of children who dislike school, and avoid it whenever possible, is probably more than five per cent of the school age population; but less than one per cent could be genuinely called school phobic. The Royal College of Psychiatrists suggests that between five and ten per cent of children and young people have anxiety problems bad enough to affect their ability to live a normal life.

This book gives information and advice to parents and carers of, and professionals working with, children aged 5 to 16 who suffer from anxiety disorders, especially separation anxiety and social phobia that are part of school phobia (see Chapter Two). Chapter One includes photocopiable pages for professionals, and parents and carers, to give to teachers to help them understand the anxieties some children have about school.

Occasionally, a child who has suffered from school phobia in primary school has it recur in secondary school, often in a different form. This book helps parents, carers and professionals support children of any age to recover from school phobia, guard against recurrence, and guard against it starting with a younger sibling. It also has many practical tips.

My interest in writing this book is largely personal. My own daughter suffered severely from school phobia, starting just before her sixth birthday and coming through about nine months later. She suffered most of the symptoms mentioned in this book and became a sickly child from constant stress and lack of food. Her ability to function outside the confines of her home became extremely limited and her fears affected her whole life, which affected ours. During the extremes of her suffering, she attended school only part time on health grounds.

I found out that most of the people I turned to for help did not know how to give it. Some were unwilling to even try. As one who likes to problem-solve, I worked hard at finding my own solutions and had these confirmed by my daughter and the child and adolescent psychiatrist to whom she was referred after persistent requests. The practical advice given in this book has come from my own experiences with my daughter.

It was only when I heard of other children suffering from school phobia that I realised it was a more common problem than I'd thought and I wanted to share what I had learnt with others to limit the damage to all involved, but most particularly to the children vulnerable in their distress.

The reasons for school phobia to play a part in any child's life are varied but the theme that is common to all is stress that the child is unable to handle. The quickest way through is to remove the stress, allowing the child to relearn that the things he or she now perceives as dangerous are completely safe. If this is not possible, the child must be helped to deal with the stress and understand why he or she has such fears and learn to keep them under control.

The stresses in my own daughter's life that led to school phobia were the following:

- We had moved to a 12th-century castle to be houseparents to students that lived in that part of the college. The building was noisy with wind, doors banging, voices echoing in corridors, flag pole wire banging against the pole, the college rescue services' call-out siren (which was an old World War II siren sited above my daughter's bedroom), fire alarms (there was a beeper in my daughter's bedroom) and doorbells on both floors of our accommodation (one of which was fixed to my daughter's bedroom door).

- Drizzle, fog, flies, wind blowing in particles and detector faults continually set off the over-sensitive fire alarms. Consequently, my daughter became very afraid of fire, of alarms, of being burnt, of going to sleep and of being left alone.

- My daughter heard students' footsteps coming up the stone stairs and was afraid someone would come into her room. (Strangers had wandered into our flat more than once to look around, having ignored all the private signs at the gates.) Consequently, my daughter became very afraid of strangers coming in, being burgled and, again, of going to sleep and of being left alone.

- Her bedroom had large shadows from the various arches and doorways and this made her afraid of things lurking in the dark.

- She had a bad bout of croup and vomited before and during her journey to hospital in the ambulance. She developed a fear of being sick, of being ill and of dying.

- There were three deaths she knew of before her trouble started and another, a friend of her father's, later in the year. This increased her fear of illness and dying.

- For some time she had an undetected urine infection that made her need to frequently visit the toilet. She worried about needing to go when there wasn't a toilet. For a year after her infection had cleared up she continued to go to the toilet with great frequency, especially when she was anxious. (This was the last symptom of her anxiety to go.)

- She stepped in dog mess one morning before getting onto the school bus and it made her feel sick. She connected vomiting in the ambulance with being sick on the school bus and was afraid to travel on the bus again.

- She was sent home from school three times as soon as she arrived because teachers thought she was ill, but she was just anxious. This increased her concern for her health, refusing to believe me when I told her she was fine.

The combined effect of these events made my daughter anxious about leaving home and not being in the same room as either my husband or me when at home, needing to follow us everywhere.

Nine months later she was a different child, having 90 per cent recovered. It helped that the student house in the castle closed and we were moved to be houseparents to students who lived adjacent to our new family house, but she had started to recover six months before. The move had just speeded up her recovery. She did briefly regress three years later but all was resolved within three weeks and this prompted me to write Chapter Nine.

Just because a child is shy or anxious about some things or situations, it is important not to label his or her whole character as such. There can be many facets to a child. For example, my daughter remains a shy child with new adults but is outgoing with friends and people she knows well. She developed an early taste for scary theme park rides on which many of her friends could not contemplate going. There are other glimpses of a determined and fun-loving personality that we try to build on, trying not to be over-protective and encouraging her to be continually challenged so that she is moving forward, but without pressurising her. We show our expectation that she will be fine. If she expresses a desire to do something, and it is within our power to agree (without there being concrete reasons to disagree), she is encouraged to go for it.

Author's note

Although professionals use the term school refusal, and sometimes school avoidance, throughout this book this condition has been referred to as school phobia. This is to avoid confusing truancy with an anxiety problem, and because many parents and carers think of a child as having school phobia, discuss the problem with others using this term and, in using it, the underlying fear the child has is immediately understood.

A chapter has been included on general information about anxiety, as school phobia is a result of extreme anxiety in children and is a complex disorder. Many anxiety disorders coexist or are linked in some way.

Because anxiety is such a big problem for children with Asperger syndrome, and many children with it experience a high degree of school phobia, information that is specific to understanding and helping these children through their particular fears has also been included. Children with Asperger syndrome need to be handled differently to children without; for example, desensitisation (graduated exposure) may cause further distress in an Asperger child yet can help a child without the syndrome.

However, it is accepted that children with AD(H)D (attention deficit (hyperactivity) disorder) and other conditions such as learning disabilities are also more prone to anxiety and anxiety disorders. Part of this may be because of having to deal with their condition, often in an environment where the people around them do not understand their difficulties or because they have not had their condition diagnosed and so are not on the road to help. Some children do not neatly fit into any one category as many have more than one condition, thus professionals may be reluctant to make any firm diagnosis at all which means the child cannot be statemented with special educational needs. Or professionals may be reluctant to look further after applying one label to a child, which can also mean that the child does not get appropriate help. Part of the difficulty in diagnosis is that children with, for example, AD(H)D have symptoms that overlap with the symptoms of other conditions including Asperger syndrome. Like children with Asperger syndrome, children with AD(H)D can have problems with social skills, making friends and co-ordination, so some of the advice given to adults dealing with anxiety in children with Asperger syndrome is also applicable to AD(H)D children (such as helping with improving the child's social skills).

Whatever the reason for a child's anxiety, this book will help adults involved with the child understand the havoc that anxiety can wreak and the distress it causes the sufferer, so that they are more tolerant and can assist the child in coping with his or her anxieties.

Chronic fatigue syndrome (CFS) – also known as myalgic encephalomyelitis (ME) – in children is often confused with anxiety or school phobia and parents and carers of children with CFS have often been accused of enabling them to truant by professionals who do not understand the condition or cannot make a diagnosis of what is wrong with the child. Because of this, children with CFS have also been mentioned.

To avoid the continual use of he/she in this book, 'she' has been used to encompass both sexes except in sections that refer to autistic spectrum disorders as this difficulty mainly occurs in boys. And to avoid the continual use of parent/carer, the word parent has been used to mean any adult who is in the position of being the main carer for the child. This person may be her natural birth parent, her adoptive or foster parent, an adult that looks after children in care or another relative such as a grandparent. When the word parents is used, this may mean either a couple or one person who has responsibility for the child.

All the web addresses listed in this book were checked prior to publishing. As time goes on, the list will become inaccurate although the addresses for organisations are not likely to change.

Chapter One

School Phobia

School phobia is not a true 'phobia'. It is far more complex and can involve a range of disorders including separation anxiety, agoraphobia and social phobia, although the anxiety is centred around the school environment. In reality, the school phobic child is usually afraid of leaving the secure home environment, and the safe presence of the main carers.

A young child suffering from separation anxiety may suffer the same symptoms when being left at a friend's home as being left at school. A child suffering from agoraphobia may suffer the same symptoms in a cinema as on the school bus. And another child, suffering from social phobia, might have the same symptoms when asked to read aloud in a place of worship, for example; so it is not only the school that causes these distressing symptoms.

However, since these symptoms of distress occur so regularly around the school environment, it is not always clear what is causing the child's turmoil and the child may be so severely affected that she cannot attend school; the general condition is conveniently termed school phobia. Some professionals prefer to call this school refusal or school avoidance but, again, confusion can come about if people think that this includes truants who experience no anxiety about school and who feel no guilt or anxiety for not having attended.

Is the child truanting?

School phobia is an umbrella term for children who do not want to go to school because of anxiety and their anxiety keeps them at home. This is contrasted with truanting children who intentionally do not go to school and who usually do not stay at home (and truanting older adolescents often show anti-social behaviour, such as being involved in criminal activities).[1] Other children may simply prefer to be at home playing, finding it more interesting than being in school and so try to get their parents' permission to be at home, but also do not experience fear.

School phobic children who do not attend school because their symptoms are so severe are not truants, because they have a specific anxiety about school and they remain at home with their parents' knowledge and, perhaps, presence. These children are children with special needs and should be dealt with in a sensitive and caring way as they are likely to be very sensitive and timid, feeling afraid of being perceived as failures.[2]

The types of school phobia

There are two types of school phobia.[3] The first is related to separation anxiety (see Chapter Four) and is generally found in children up to age eight (although older children can suffer from this too: the longer separation anxiety continues, the more difficult it is to treat). The younger child is less likely to have learnt to feel confident and to be independent away from her parents. The onset of separation anxiety is usually sudden in children who have had it naturally subside after the age of three[1] although it can start from the age of six to eight months and continue thereafter.

The second type predominantly affects children above age eight and revolves around the social aspects of the school and can be considered to be social phobia (see Chapter Five). The onset of this is gradual and can start from increased self-awareness around the time of puberty.[4]

Sometimes, travelling to school is the problem; the child may suffer from agoraphobia (see Chapter Two). However, this is usually an extension of other anxiety problems the child has and so it would probably also be present in a child who has separation anxiety. The child may want her parents to drive her to school, fearing that something embarrassing might happen on the bus or train, and not feeling secure unless with someone to look after her should she feel panicky. (This was the case with my daughter, who feared being sick on the school bus, relating it to the times she'd been sick in the ambulance and when she'd felt sick on the school bus after stepping in dog mess.)

Three age groups that have peaks in school phobia

There are three peaks for school phobia:[1,2]

- The first is at age five to seven, and is related to separation anxiety.

- The second predominates at age 11 to 12, due to the anxieties associated with changing from a primary to a secondary school, and is linked to social phobia.

- The third is at age 14 to 16 and is linked to social phobia and other psychiatric disorders such as depression and other phobias.

There may be another small peak due to separation anxiety when children have a change in school building when they move from infants to juniors, or from first to middle schools at age seven to eight. Fears children have when starting or changing school usually develop in the early months of the first term, typically September to November in the northern hemisphere. Separation anxiety can be exacerbated by a return to school after holidays.

Indicators of susceptibility in children

There are certain family characteristics[1] that indicate whether a child is likely to be more susceptible to suffering an anxiety disorder such as school phobia. Indicators are:

- Another close family member suffers from an emotional or anxiety-related problem.

- The child has been over-protected and is therefore often more dependent on her parents, fearful of going it alone. (This is possibly the case with an only child.)

- The child has a very anxious mother, and the mother's anxiety is transmitted to the child, making her feel that she also has cause to worry. (The child can also 'model' her mother, and behave in the same way that her mother does, worrying about the same sort of things in the same sort of way.)

- The child may have a father who plays little part in her upbringing or he may be absent altogether.

- The youngest child in a family is often the most vulnerable to anxiety disorders because she is considered always to be the 'baby' of the family and is treated as such. Also, when parents know they will have no more children, they sometimes want to keep the youngest very close to them and, albeit unconsciously, dependent.

- The child has a chronic illness and has needed to be very dependent on her parents and has not had the confidence to know she is fit and strong and able to cope with what life throws at her.

- The child is often well behaved and academically able.

School phobia can develop as the result of depression[1], which makes the child feel she can't possibly cope with the pressures and challenges of school or as the result of an escalation of a number of fears and stressors (as with my daughter).

The symptoms of school phobia
Whatever anxiety disorder or disorders the child is suffering from, she can experience anxiety symptoms including:
- crying
- diarrhoea
- feeling faint
- a frequent need to urinate
- headaches
- hyperventilation

- insomnia
- nausea and vomiting
- a rapid heartbeat
- shaking
- stomachaches
- sweating.

School phobic children feel very unwell when having to go to school. The symptoms disappear once the 'threat' of going to school is lifted. For example, once a child has convinced a parent that she really is ill this time and the parent gives the child the benefit of the doubt, the child relaxes and the symptoms fade. However, they return as soon as the 'threat' is reintroduced.

How does school phobia start?

Going to school for the first time is a period of great anxiety for very young children. Many will be separated from their parents for the first time, or will be separated all day for the first time. This sudden change can make them anxious and they may suffer from separation anxiety. They are also probably unused to having the entire day organised for them and may be very tired by the end of the day, causing further stress and making them feel very vulnerable.

For older children who are not new to the school, who have had a long summer break or have had time off because of illness, returning to school can be quite traumatic. They may no longer feel at home there. Their friendships may have changed. Their teacher and classroom may have changed. They may have got used to being at home and closely looked after by a parent, feeling insecure when all this attention is removed and suddenly they are under the scrutiny of their teachers again.

Other children may have felt unwell on the school bus or in school and associate these places with further illness and symptoms of panic, and so want to avoid them in order to avoid panicky symptoms and panic attacks fearing, for example, vomiting, fainting or having diarrhoea. Other children may have experienced stressful events.

Possible triggers for school phobia (collected from literature mentioned at the end of the chapter) include:

1. Being bullied.

2. Starting school for the first time.

3. Moving to a new area and having to start at a new school and make new friends, or just changing schools.

4. Being off school for a long time through illness or because of a holiday.

5. Bereavement (of a person or pet).

6. Feeling threatened by the arrival of a new baby.

7. Having a traumatic experience such as being abused, being raped or having witnessed a tragic event.

8. Problems at home such as a member of the family being very ill.

9. Problems at home such as marital rows, separation and divorce.

10. Violence in the home or any kind of abuse, of the child or of another parent.

11. Not having good friends (or any friends at all).

12. Being unpopular, being chosen last for teams and feeling a physical failure (in games and gymnastics).

13. Feeling an academic failure.

14. Fearing panic attacks when travelling to school or while in school.

(Please note that depression has not been included here as a cause of school phobia, as its potential underlying reasons have been covered in the points above.)

- Point 1 is looked at in Chapter Three.

- Points 2–10 can be related to separation anxiety, where the child feels insecure away from her parents or fears that something may happen either to herself or to a parent during the period of separation. These are looked at more closely in Chapter Four.

- Points 11–13 are concerned with social performance and are looked at more closely in Chapter Five.

- Point 14 is concerned with agoraphobia and panic disorder and is looked at further in this chapter and in chapters Two and Seven, where help for specific and general fears is given.

Please note that the above points are not intended to cast blame on the child's parents. However, if a child's fears are to be addressed it often helps for the root cause or causes to be identified and in doing this, steps can be taken to help the child. It is understood that every home has its problems (including mine). Being aware of what they are and the effect they are having allows parents to look objectively at the situation to see what they can do to help the child. The main concern has to be for the child, whatever her reason for stress.

Risks of untreated school phobia

If the school phobia is so severe that the child stops going to school, her education and social development may suffer. Since school phobia in older children tends to be centred around social phobia, this withdrawal from the social aspects of school can compound the difficulties the child already has. Also, parents have the problem of finding alternative ways of educating the child (see *Home education* in Chapter Seven).

Temporary home tuition may make it harder for the child to return to school. However, children with autistic spectrum disorders may benefit hugely from a long break and may even fare better out of the school system if they do not respond well to the school environment, particularly in their teens when they may also be suffering from obsessive compulsive disorders and depression.[5] There are also special schools that specifically cater for children with autistic spectrum disorders (see below).

Although permanent removal from mainstream education may make the child happier, professionals are concerned that if a child's underlying fears have never been addressed and dealt with, the child may store up problems for the future. For example, the child may fear leaving home to go to college or work, the previously unresolved fears holding her back, making her very dependent on family support. The lack of social contact may also have a detrimental effect, making it hard for her to make friends in a new environment and be socially on the same wavelength as the majority. And, if the child is already very shy or over-sensitive, she is more likely to remain so.

Once the child's anxieties interfere with her everyday life, parents should seek help from a child and adolescent mental health professional such as a child psychologist or psychiatrist.

Special schools for children with autistic spectrum disorders

Children with autistic spectrum disorders who attend special schools may have fewer of the problems such children face in mainstream schools because the environment is adapted to suit their particular needs.

Jayne Birch, Headteacher of Springhallow (Ealing, London), a special school for children with autistic spectrum disorders, says:

> I do think specialist education is often the best place to assist anxious pupils with autistic spectrum disorders (ASD). I often visit pupils with ASD who are placed in mainstream schools and they find the whole experience stressful, confusing and scary. Our older pupils who have been with us since they were small are not overly anxious and none have developed obsessive compulsive disorders. The pupils who cause us most concern in these areas are those who have come from/been excluded from mainstream schools as older pupils. They are often distressed and take a long time to build relationships. They often have high anxiety levels.
>
> Our environment is ordered and structured, calm and quiet, even when pupils and staff move around the school. Lunchtimes and assemblies too have a routine and are well staffed. Our teaching styles are designed to assist the pupils in managing their anxiety: we break things into small manageable tasks. Much anxiety is caused by pupils not knowing what is going to happen next, needing to control their environment and often not being able to, and wanting reassurance and confidence boosters. We also teach our pupils (from a very early age) how to calm themselves and how to ask for help. Calmness is the key to managing and working with pupils with ASD and most of our pupils do not need breaks because of anxiety.

Is it school phobia? Identifying the cause of the child's symptoms

Symptoms of school phobia have already been mentioned. However, it is important not to label the child as school phobic until other causes of her symptoms have been considered.

Is the child tired?

Is the child getting enough sleep? Does she go to bed early enough? If she can't get to sleep at night, is she having sufficient exercise? Is she eating enough to fuel her needs? The child's doctor should be consulted if the parent has concerns about her diet. The child might be growing so fast that she has no energy left for anything else. Or she might be anaemic or her doctor might consider having her tested for glandular fever.

Has the child done her homework?

Was the child supposed to give something in that she hasn't done? Does she fear getting into trouble because of it? If parents check her homework diary (if she has one) each day, they will know what is outstanding.

What exactly are the child's physical symptoms?

Getting a clearer picture of what is physically wrong helps parents come to a decision. A vague stomachache may go. If the child is rarely ill (or never suffers from indefinite symptoms without later apparent illness) and she is very young, parents may decide to give her the benefit of the doubt and keep her at home for observation. If she is older, parents may tell the child that her stomachache may go and send her to school.

Vague symptoms that do not prevent the child from eating her breakfast are not usually sufficient reason to keep her home from school, unless she has a history of illnesses starting in this way. However, if parents are concerned, they should take the child to her doctor to be checked out. If it turns out to be nothing, it may help allay her anxiety. (My own daughter had stomachache that came and went: it later turned out she had a urine infection.)

Does the child like her teacher?

Try to remember all that the child has said about her teacher. Was she shouted at the previous day? Had she been in trouble over something? Is there an ongoing problem? Is her teacher going to be absent and the child dislikes the replacement teacher?

Is the teacher causing a problem?

Is the child being picked on by a teacher or being abused in some way? Parents should closely question her if they suspect this and must be careful not to lay any blame on the child. Does the teacher use non-professional methods such as deliberately poking fun at children who make mistakes, making a public example of them or calling them unkind names? Is the teacher deliberately insensitive as a form of class control? Does the teacher increase hostilities between children or groups of children in the class by what he or she says (such as by openly identifying intelligent or academically challenged children)?

Is there anything different about the day?

Is the child anxious about a school trip that's going to take place? Is the format of the day going to change in some other way? Does she have a test? Will her best friend be away? Is there one particular teacher she tries to avoid? (And if so, why?)

Is there a problem in getting to school?

Does the child dislike going on the school bus (or on public transport)? Is she picked on while going to school? (If this were to happen on a school bus there may be a 'helper' who takes charge of the children whom she or her parents could tell.)

Does the child have friendship problems?

Does the child have friends? Is she being bullied?

Is the child trying it on?

Children like to test boundaries and, as they get older, they retest to move the boundaries further and further back. Is the child trying it on to see if her parents will give in? There may be no more to it than her fancying a day off school and pretending to be ill. And if she succeeds once, she will be sure to try again.

Is the child using her reluctance as a weapon?

If parents have something special planned for the day that the child knows about, would she deliberately try to spoil it by being off school and needing their presence at home? Is she exacting revenge? Has the relationship lately been marred by something?

Is the child attention seeking?

The child may fancy a day at home being cuddled by her parents. Have the child's parents encouraged her to seek attention by giving in too easily to her demands?

Is the child overloaded with work?

Has the child got behind with her commitments? Is she too busy after school and at the weekends to fulfil her academic commitments or is she lacking in organisational skills? The child may feel that her work is getting on top of her. If the child's work needs to be rescheduled, parents could discuss it with the teacher concerned or write a note to her teacher in her homework diary. They should help the child make time to do it. Being off school in order to catch up puts other demands on her. She needs to learn to plan ahead so that this doesn't happen. Perhaps a chunk of the weekend (such as Saturday morning) could be devoted to homework alone.

Is the child having difficulties with her work?

Does the child have special educational needs, or do her parents think that she needs to be assessed (she might be dyslexic, for example)? Many children suffer anxiety about being in school, because they find the work too hard and this is a demoralising experience. Parents need to make sure that the child gets any help she needs, whether a little extra tuition at home with her teacher guiding the parents, or from a special needs teacher.

If none of the above possibilities apply to the child, and she has extreme anxiety about attending school or travelling to school, she probably has school phobia. When a child is anxious, it may be very difficult to pin down the cause of her anxiety or to understand what is happening to her. Parents may not fully understand what has gone wrong until long after her recovery. (I hadn't managed to string everything together until up to a year after my daughter's recovery. Then it seemed obvious. Researching and writing this book further helped my understanding.)

Parents must support the child as she will undoubtedly be suffering, the symptoms of anxiety and panic being uncomfortable and frightening for her. They may be the only ones on her 'side', particularly if her teachers are unsympathetic. Also, parents should understand that what is happening to the child is not something she can snap out of. Children do not deliberately make themselves ill and cut themselves off from social contact the school environment provides.

Parents should reassure the child and show they understand how she feels, without criticising her for being so inadequate as not to be able to cope with the simple matter of going to school. They should not make her feel a failure because she cannot 'pull herself together' but give her permission to have these feelings and encourage her to talk about them so that they have some idea about what is going on in her head. Also, parents should try to relax expectations of the child for as long as necessary; some things just don't matter and the child may need a break from all negative input from home.

If the child suffers extreme distress about going to school and it is not resolved in a few weeks, parents will need to seek professional help.

Other reasons why children refuse school

This section looks at two problems many children face that affect their ability to cope with school. The first is autistic spectrum disorders where children (mostly boys) can experience extreme anxiety and panic attacks (and other conditions mentioned in Chapter Two); the second is chronic fatigue syndrome (CFS), sometimes known as myalgic encephalomyelitis (ME).

Refusing school: children with autistic spectrum disorders

The problems children with high-functioning autism and Asperger syndrome face are not related to intelligence (they are usually of average or above-average intelligence) but particular impairments (called the 'triad of impairments') that hinder their ability to make sense of the world.[6] These children may not have all the impairments but all have some of them, the particular mix being individual to the child. The child must have impairments in all three areas for a diagnosis of Asperger syndrome or autism to be made. Impairments seen in only two out of three areas will lead to a diagnosis, for example, of atypical autism or pervasive development disorder not otherwise specified.

PROBLEMS WITH SOCIAL COMMUNICATION

Children with high-functioning autism and Asperger syndrome:

- Find it hard to understand and use: gestures (pointing, 'come here', waving), postures (why they should sit up straight in class but can slouch at home), facial expressions (angry, happy, sad, pleased) and voice information (pitch, tone, speed). They may also have difficulty in making eye contact.

- Find it hard to communicate with their peers (communication with adults is easier as they are more predictable and are more likely to be able to anticipate their needs).[7] This leads to social isolation and a lack of motivation in wanting to interact with their peers (even though many do want to be able to socialise),[8] as they don't find the experience rewarding if they get ridiculed and rejected. This can lead to anxiety in social situations (even social phobia) and nervous tics (involuntary sounds or movements). It also lays the children open to being bullied.

- Find it hard to express themselves, particularly how they feel.

PROBLEMS WITH SOCIAL UNDERSTANDING

Children with high-functioning autism and Asperger syndrome:

- Find it hard to choose topics to talk about or to make other decisions. However, they may talk incessantly about topics that are of special interest to them regardless of whether the listener is interested.

- Take what is said literally and are unable to interpret jokes, double meanings, idioms and teasing.

- Find making small talk hard (they don't see the point of it).

- Are unaware of why some topics of conversation are unsuitable (for example, understanding that there are taboo subjects or that topics of conversation they can have with their friends are different to those they can have with adults).

- Have difficulty in group situations (for example, not understanding that they should wait their turn or that they should not interrupt someone else).

PROBLEMS WITH IMAGINATION AND INNER LANGUAGE

Children with high-functioning autism and Asperger syndrome can have impairments of their imagination (this does not refer to creative ability, which they can have in abundance): visualising alternative outcomes and predicting what might happen next. Consequently, they may:

- Find it hard to take part in imaginative play such as taking the roles of different people or imagining that a tree house is a space ship.

- Have trouble in understanding how other people are feeling or what they are thinking.

- Find it hard to predict what will happen next, such as in a story or when on a trip.

- Find it hard to organise their life (such as understanding the sequencing of tasks necessary for getting ready for school or what they need to take with them) or make plans for a future event.

Children with high-functioning autism and Asperger syndrome also often have problems linked to dyspraxia,[8, 9] which is a difficulty in planning and carrying out sensory/motor tasks, presenting difficulties in handwriting (fine motor impairment) and clumsiness, tripping and falling (gross motor impairment). They may also have sensitivity to smell, light, sound, touch and taste.[10]

Any child who is anxious about being in school due to the unpredictability of the day and the fear of ridicule and rejection will have problems learning. But a child who also has to contend with laughters over clumsy behaviour and social rejection because of not fitting in, no matter how hard he tries, has additional hurdles. Treating such a child with the kindness and respect he deserves and ensuring that those around him are inclusive and understanding, tolerant of his differences and his need sometimes to be quiet and alone, might allow him access to education among his peers that he has every right to expect.

Nothing should be forced on a child with an autistic spectrum disorder as his anxiety is at a high level anyway. The key to including such a child and allowing him to progress in his social awareness and motor skills is to provide an environment that can accommodate his differences so that he can make use of what's on offer.

Refusing school: children with CFS

CFS (chronic fatigue syndrome), ME (myalgic encephalomyelitis) and CFIDS (chronic fatigue immunity deficiency syndrome) are names doctors use to describe the debilitating fatigue and other symptoms sufferers experience. Although the cause of the illness can vary, it often follows a viral infection from which the sufferer has been unable to completely recover. For the purpose of easy description, this illness shall be referred to in this book as CFS since this is the term most used by professionals.

In children, CFS has often been confused with school phobia or parental collusion with the child staying at home, the child's genuine symptoms not being taken seriously. A child suffering from the debilitating illness of CFS does not have school phobia.

HOW DO I KNOW IF THE CHILD HAS CFS?

The main symptom is complete exhaustion, often to the point of collapse. Sufferers often feel nauseous and faint or dizzy. A child with CFS will often need to sit down, finding standing impossible because of faintness and tiredness. She may have poor short-term memory, have difficulty finding the right words to use and difficulty thinking clearly. Her balance may also be affected, being unable to walk in a straight line. She may have headaches and pains in her muscles, and suffer from insomnia even though she is dreadfully tired.

Some sufferers are also sensitive to light and noise and can become extremely sensitive to medication or certain foods. Other symptoms may also be present. The number of symptoms a child has, and their severity, can be individual to the child.[11]

Before a clinical diagnosis of CFS can be made, the possibility of other illnesses needs to be ruled out; thus, a positive diagnosis can take some time. However, once a diagnosis has been made, it is vital that the child is not pushed to do more than she can cope with, as this prolongs the illness and can make it worse.

Some children may be able to attend school with help and support (being taken to and from school, being excused from all sport, being able to sit down or rest at break times), while others are unable to do anything for themselves without assistance.

Sometimes, after the child has been ill for a long time and is ready to attend school for short periods each day or for a morning once or twice a week, the anxiety that this causes may make the child unable to face going back to school. Unsympathetic staff and peers can make her return intolerable. She may even be bullied.

It is vital that staff and peers understand that CFS is a real illness and how devastating it is to the sufferer. One of the biggest hurdles a sufferer of CFS has to face is disbelief in others: people thinking that the child is feigning illness. This isolates the child from support and understanding and can lead to depression. She needs to know that there are people on her side, willing to support her, understanding her needs and difficulties. She needs to know that they'll understand if she has a relapse and has to be absent from school again for a few weeks, or that they are prepared to be flexible, working around her everyday needs. Lack of sympathy in dealing with the child will only make her fear going to school and destroy her faith in humanity.

Parents can get support and information from one of the CFS groups mentioned in *Useful Contacts*, from their local library and the Internet. Being informed, and being able to take evidence of the child's symptoms to the child's doctor, will help understanding.

Try to empathise with the school phobic child

It is often hard for teachers and other professionals who work with children to understand why a child is so scared; teachers in particular, understandably want the school environment to be seen as a safe, friendly place. Thus, to empathise with the child, teachers should try to imagine their greatest fears and how they would feel if they had to face them day after day and, to make matters worse, with many people being unhelpful because they do not understand. It would probably make them feel powerless, out of control, angry, hurt, terribly stressed and vulnerable.

The child probably lives those fears every minute, even when she gets home, as she knows there will be school the following day or the following Monday. Her dreams will be taken up with her fears. She may have trouble getting to sleep, be frightened of the dark and relive her greatest nightmare again the moment she wakes up.

Unless her teachers know what it is to be so frightened or stressed that they have vomited, had diarrhoea and felt a constant urge to urinate, they may not be able to appreciate what the child has to face in coming to school. She needs comfort, reassurance and some sort of acknowledgement for the desperate struggle within her, for being so brave in simply turning up to school, let alone staying there all day.

If the child's teachers can make the child's time in class non-threatening, rewarding and reassuring, the child may relax enough to take in some of the lesson. Schools that are highly evaluative and authoritarian can provide increased stress for the child and make her feel demoralised and more helpless than ever. It is well known that children under stress cannot learn effectively.

It may be useful to photocopy the previous pages to give to the child's class teacher and/or Head of Year, to help him or her understand

School Phobia

School phobia is often known as school refusal or school avoidance because it is not a 'true' phobia. It is far more complex and can include a range of disorders including separation anxiety, agoraphobia and social phobia, although the child's anxiety is centred on the school environment. Some school phobic children are depressed.

School phobic children who are frequently absent from school are not truants, because children who truant experience no anxiety about attending school and, when they 'bunk off', don't tend to stay at home, but are out all day. School phobic children, when not in school, are relieved to be in the safety of their home with their main carers. School phobic children can suffer anxiety symptoms that include:

- crying

- diarrhoea

- feeling faint

- a frequent need to urinate

- headaches

- hyperventilation

- insomnia

- nausea and vomiting

- a rapid heartbeat

- stomachaches

- shaking

- sweating.

Spending many hours each day feeling anxious, and not getting sufficient refreshing sleep, can take its toll on the school phobic child. She* will probably feel very tired all the

* 'She' has been used to avoid the clumsy use of 'he/she'.

time. She may also feel low or depressed because of feeling so horrible. It can therefore not be stressed enough that she needs to be handled with great care and gentleness: it may have a great bearing on her future.

A child suffering from school phobia is not attention seeking, or spoilt or encouraged to stay at home by her main carers. A child who has school phobia cannot 'snap out of it' or 'pull herself together'. No previously co-operative and well behaved child would willingly deny herself the pleasure of becoming fully involved with the school environment and friends. The child does not gain from being school phobic, but loses.

There can be many triggers of separation anxiety such as: starting school for the first time; being absent for a long time due to ill health or a holiday; having a new baby in the family who makes the child feel threatened; suffering bereavement; having troubles at home; or being bullied. For some children, there may be no obvious cause.

Older children, from age eight upward and particularly adolescents, can suffer from social phobia but may also have separation anxiety. Social phobia is a fear of being judged and evaluated by others, and children that suffer from it may seem aloof, awkward, backward, disinterested, inhibited, nervous, quiet, shy, unfriendly and withdrawn. Despite wanting to make friends and become involved, they are hampered by their anxiety. In school they will fear being the centre of attention: having to answer or read aloud in class; being involved in assemblies, performances, games lessons and sports day; being picked last for teams; and having others laughing at their mistakes or ineptitude.

The best way for teachers to approach a child suffering from anxiety is to deal with her very sensitively (she is very vulnerable at this time) and show her that they care about her and are on her side.

Dos

- Do let the child visit the toilet as often as she wants. She may need to wee or vomit or she may have diarrhoea. The child should never be prevented from going to the toilet and it helps if she is not made to feel embarrassed by needing to go so often or she will feel more ill at ease and uncomfortable in school. Let her go without fuss or attention directed her way.

- Do praise the child whenever possible to make school a rewarding place to be.

- Do praise all the children within the class whenever possible so that the child is taught in a positive and rewarding environment.

- Do always treat the child with consideration and respect.

- Do lower expectations (this is not favouritism: it is acknowledgement of a disability less obvious perhaps than that of other children). For example, she may not want to join in with PE or read out loud in class or perform in assembly. She should never be forced to do something that will increase her tension or be made to feel embarrassed in front of her peers.

- Do think carefully about what is said to the child, as she will be hypersensitive to any form of criticism, real or perceived. A great deal of damage may be done by the odd careless remark, undoing weeks of confidence boosting by her main carers. The slightest negative comment can have big repercussions and the child may withdraw further into herself and distrust her teacher.

- Do acknowledge the effort it takes for a school phobic child to attend school, and the distress it causes in the family. Show pleasure that she has managed to come to school.

- Do explain a young child's problem to others in the class in a basic and matter-of-fact way so that they become more understanding and tolerant. This may help her be socially accepted, as the other children see the problem as a recognised medical condition. (Teachers should discuss it with the child's main carers first and ask the child's permission, explaining why they think it may help.) Older children who are social phobic will not want more attention drawn to them so will probably refuse permission for this to happen. However, they may appreciate their very close friends being told about their condition as they may have difficulty explaining it themselves.

- Do intervene immediately if there is any suggestion of bullying behaviour. Explain why it is not acceptable. The child needs to be protected from all negative experiences and she needs to feel a part of the school, not further isolated or ridiculed.

- Do try to anticipate the child's needs and smooth over her fears, particularly if it is known beforehand that the child will find a forthcoming event hard.

- Do create an environment where the child can be successful. If she is slow with her work, for example, give the class plenty of warning before the bell goes for the end of the lesson by counting down every 5 minutes from 15 minutes to the bell. Give her work in bite-sized pieces and keep checking she understands what she's meant to be doing. This can be done covertly by wandering around the class looking at all the children's progress or by crouching beside her and talking quietly to her as well as other children (so that she does not feel singled out).

- Do try to include the child in group activities, as social isolation will compound her problems (unless she has a specific condition like Asperger syndrome where this could increase her anxiety). If the group she is in is small and stays the same, she will feel safe and included within the group.

- Do comfort a primary school phobic child. If the child is very young, she may appreciate being met at the gate or in the class the moment she comes in, as this will be the highest stress point of her day. The sooner she calms down, the sooner she will be more receptive to what is going on around her. She needs to know that her teacher can care for her and that she is safe with him or her.

- Do identify a special contact person (a mentor) for a secondary school phobic child. This may be the form teacher or the Head of Year or a special needs teacher. It is important that the child feels there is someone there for her that she can turn to who cares about her well being. She may appreciate going to this person when she arrives.

- Do inform all teachers with whom the child is likely to be in contact about her problem and give appropriate advice so that they, too, can make the child's experience of their interaction rewarding without drawing unwelcome attention to the child.

- Do let the child be educated in the special unit (if the school has one) if she has severe problems. Some children may have to give up attending school altogether because their symptoms are so severe. The special unit acts as a halfway house between home and full mainstream schooling. As soon as the child is ready she can be re-integrated into the classroom with her peers. The advantage of the special unit is that it more closely resembles the cosiness and security of the child's home. Only when the child feels secure is she going to be calm enough to gain from being in school.

Don'ts

- Don't send the child home if she complains of feeling ill without first verifying her symptoms, so that she is not sent home unnecessarily. (Otherwise the child will be convinced she is ill when she's not, mistaking her panic symptoms for those of genuine illness.) However, a child who is genuinely unwell, showing some symptoms that aren't anxiety-related (such as a raised temperature), should not be kept in school.

- Don't punish the child because she does not conform to the behaviour of others in the class; it is not her fault and she cannot help it. An example of an unhelpful comment might be, 'I'm disappointed you didn't come on the school bus with the rest of your class. Isn't it good enough for you?'

- Don't apportion blame to the child or her main carers (even if they blame the school). It is unhelpful if teachers feel they need to make it clear that it is not a school problem. It is most definitely a school problem even if teachers feel the trigger is not attributable to the school.

- Don't make a joke at the expense of the child. She will feel humiliated and the joke may well be continued in the schoolyard.

- Don't say any negative things to the child about herself or her behaviour.

- Don't ignore the child's hand if it is raised for the very first time. She needs to be rewarded for taking such a positive step. If it is to answer a question that turns out to be right, praise her lavishly. If the answer she gives is wrong, explain to the class why it was an understandable mistake to make so that the child does not feel she failed altogether.

- Don't let the pupils choose their teams for games if the child is unpopular as this will make her feel worse about herself, particularly if she is always chosen last.

- Don't force her to take part in sports day or to go on school trips and don't make her feel bad about not attending on those days.

In term time children spend most of their time in school, so if they find it an unrewarding and frightening place to be it can have a big negative impact on their lives, causing immense distress and suffering, affecting their physical and mental health. School phobia is a difficult problem for a child to recover from, but with the child's teachers and main carers working together, there is a much better chance that the child's problems will be short-lived and that the severity of the child's unpleasant physical symptoms will be much reduced.

the nature of the child's problems, what he or she can do to help, and what things are unhelpful.

Conclusion

A school phobic child is basically a child who has lost all confidence in herself and one who feels very insecure and scared. In order to redress the balance, every opportunity of giving the child a rewarding experience should be taken so that her self-confidence is raised. Being rewarded is addictive. Children like to repeat the experience, so there is no reason why, if the child is regularly rewarded in school even for the most basic things, she might not start to see it in a more positive light and feel a successful and valued part of that school.

The child's new found confidence in school will turn around the fearful and insecure feelings she has, taking her on the road to recovery and allowing her to resume a 'normal' life. The role of a helping adult in the child's life at this time is an enormous and responsible one. She needs to see that she is valued and understood so that she can have confidence in the adults who care for her and believe that school is a good place to be.

References

1. www.mcevoy.demon.co.uk/medicine/psychiatry/
    childpsych/school.html

2. www.anxietycare.org.uk/documents/child.html

3. National Phobics Society (see *Useful Contacts*) factsheet on school phobia.

4. www.anxietycare.org.uk/documents.social.html

5. Attwood, T. (1998) *Asperger's Syndrome: A Guide for Parents and Professionals.* London: Jessica Kingsley Publishers, p.156.

6. www.nas.org.uk/pubs/faqs/qaddiag.html#describing

7. www.autism-uk.ed.ac.uk/advice.html

8. www.udel.edu/bkirby/asperger/aswhatisit.html

9. www.ratbag.demon.co.uk/anna/asa/definitions/sensory.html

10. Attwood, T. (1998) *Asperger's Syndrome: A Guide for Parents and Professionals.* London: Jessica Kingsley Publishers, pp.129–140.

11. www.westcareuk.org.uk

Further reading

Information and advice on school phobia can be found on the following webpages:

> www.mcevoy.demon.co.uk/medicine/psychiatry/childpsych/predisps.html

> www.mcevoy.demon.co.uk/medicine/psychiatry/childpsych/anxphobs/treatnprog.html

> www.artscroll.com/chapters/pwhh-015.html

> "'I don't want to go to school." Faking or phobia?' Extract from Chapter 15 from *Partners with Hashem: Effective Guidelines for Successful Parenting* by Dr Meir Wikler. Brooklyn, NY: Artscroll-Mesorah.

> www.drpaul.com/behaviour/schoolphobia.html

Information and advice on high-functioning autism and Asperger syndrome can be found on the following websites:

> www.nas.org.uk/pubs/asd/index.html (The National Autistic Society website containing information and advice on autism and Asperger syndrome.)

> www.autism-society.org (Website of the Autism Society of America containing information on autism.)

> www.udel.edu/bkirby/asperger/oasis (Online Asperger syndrome Information and Support.)

> www.aspie.org (Asperger's Syndrome Parent Information Environment website.)

> www.angelfire.com/amiga/aut (A personal website describing Asperger syndrome.)

> www.vaporia.com/autism (Information and links on autism and Asperger syndrome.)

Chapter Two

Anxiety Disorders

Anxiety can be a useful part of a child's life. Mild anxiety can drive her to achieve her full potential by making her feel threatened by competitors and by fearing failure. Adrenaline, the hormone secreted by the body when stressed, can help the child perform well in tests, firing her brain to work at top speed and it can help when she is competing on a physical level, by readying her muscles for action using her 'fight or flight' response (see below).

When in a crisis such as being in danger, anxiety can see a child through due to the 'fight or flight' mechanism her body has, which is designed to protect her by making her ready for action. But if this crisis is not dealt with in a physical way (such as by fighting or running away from the danger) because her anxiety is due to stress or a perceived threat (such as with a phobia), the physical symptoms of anxiety are not relieved. She can then become anxious about the way she is feeling, causing further anxiety. This creates a spiral of increasing anxiety known as positive feedback. (The original anxiety causes further anxiety as the child worries over her symptoms and this further anxiety increases the severity of her symptoms, making her more anxious still as her need to worry about her symptoms is, to her mind, confirmed.) If this circle is unbroken it can lead to a panic attack, which is really anxiety that has got out of the child's control.

The anxious child

If a child is over-anxious or so highly sensitive that a relatively small anxiety provokes a large response, her mind and body suffer. In fact, the anxiety can be so overwhelming that she ceases to function properly. Symptoms of anxiety can include:

- abdominal pain
- a dry mouth
- feeling faint
- frequent emptying of the bowels
- frequent urination
- nausea
- quick shallow breathing (which can lead to hyperventilation)
- rapid heartbeat
- sweating
- tense muscles.

If a child is very anxious she may worry over the slightest things that she previously took in her stride. For example, any change to the usual running of the school day might spark off anxiety, such as if her parent is supposed to collect her from school at the end of the day instead of her getting on the school bus, she may be desperately anxious about whether he or she might forget.

She might be worried about going to a club after school: she may suddenly express fears about going or say that she doesn't want to go. She might worry about having to change for sports and how she does in sports. She might worry about what she's going to be given to eat at lunchtime and whether she'll like it and with whom she'll sit. She might worry if she is away from school for a day, thinking her favourite friend may have made closer friends with someone else or that she won't know about the work she's got to do because she won't be at the same stage as her friends. Or she might be worried about her schoolwork because she doesn't understand it but everyone she sits with seems to find it easy.

Such a child is likely to be eager to please, well behaved, quiet and hard working. She may need constant reassurance that all is well and that she is doing things right.

These early signs of anxiety are the first indications that a child is in distress. If possible, parents should try to find out what the child is worrying about (suggestions were given in the previous chapter).

A child who is persistently anxious finds it harder to make and enjoy friends and relax in social situations, being too concerned about her performance. (This may affect her educational development, being too preoccupied with her private concerns to be able to concentrate.) She may put herself down and feel a failure, thinking that her parents will not love her or that she won't have friends if she cannot do better, lowering her self-esteem.

The ideal is a happy, confident child and nothing else matters when one considers the other road of panic, fear and inability to function independently of a parent. If parents cannot find out what is troubling the child and her anxiety continues, they should consider seeking professional help.

Phobias

A phobia is an irrational fear of something that is not necessarily harmful and, although the sufferer may be aware of this, she will go to great lengths to avoid the thing or situation that causes the fear. The child's reaction to the event or object is completely out of proportion to the threat that it poses. For example, a child that has a phobia of spiders (arachnophobia) knows that only a few are potentially harmful and that these only exist naturally in certain parts of the world. So screaming when she sees a small harmless spider is an exaggerated and misplaced response of fear. Children cope with phobias like this by avoiding the trigger (in this case, spiders).

There are three main categories of phobic anxiety disorders given in the *ICD-10 Classification of Mental and Behavioural Disorders* (WHO 1992): agoraphobia, social phobia and specific phobias such as arachnophobia.

Agoraphobia

Agoraphobia is common in children who suffer from panic disorder (see *Panic disorder* later in this chapter). They are anxious about being in places or situations from where they cannot escape, or from where the escape might be embarrassing, and in situations where help is not immediately available should they suddenly feel panicky. An example of this would be travelling on the school bus. Once on, the child cannot escape until the bus has reached the end of its journey. As the journey progresses, the child's mounting anxiety can trigger a panic attack. (Or even the prospect of going on the bus can trigger a panic attack.)

The agoraphobic child restricts her social life and prefers to stay at home rather than go to a friend's home or to school. She may insist that she's not well, suddenly developing a stomachache five minutes before she's due to leave, not feeling safe or secure away from home and her parents. The anxiety of being at a place from where she cannot immediately get back home can be too great for her to want to deal with. It would be embarrassing for her to have to explain to her hosts or teachers why she wants to leave early.

Any changes to the school day can make the agoraphobic child worse, such as having to go on school trips, having to take part in school performances and having a different teacher or an unexpected change in timetable.[1]

Agoraphobia and panic attacks are much more common in children who have separation anxiety (see Chapter Four: *Separation anxiety*) or have had it in the past, and all three disorders can coexist. Children who suffer either from panic attacks or from agoraphobia are much more likely to also develop the other condition (and other anxiety disorders). Depression is also common in children who suffer anxiety disorders, and the combination greatly increases the risk of suicide.[1] Agoraphobia is further mentioned in Chapter Seven.

Social phobia

Social phobia often starts in adolescence, the most predominant age of onset being between 11 and 15[2] (when children are very aware of themselves, feel very self-conscious and are over-sensitive to comments made by others), but can start in younger children from about age eight.

In young children, social phobia is often centred around school, the children feeling concerned about how they perform in front of others, the school offering the most threat to their self-confidence. In older adolescents, the fear may centre more on how well they can dance at discos, the anxiety of meeting the first boyfriend's/girlfriend's expectations, having to go to more adult functions, perhaps with parents, and eating and chatting in a formal environment where they feel out of their depth, gauche and tongue-tied. (Social phobia is looked at more closely in Chapter Five.)

Specific phobias

Specific phobias are easily defined things or events that cause extreme fear. For example, a child might be afraid of storms or birds or snakes. On the whole, these can easily be avoided, and only enforced proximity or experience of these fears causes great anxiety and panic attacks. They differ from agoraphobia and social phobia in that these have many variables. Agoraphobic or social fear depends on whom the child is with, where she is and what she has to do. One social phobic or agoraphobic child might find some things easier than another socially phobic or agoraphobic child, whereas children with specific phobias are all frightened of the same triggering factor in the same way. Examples of specific phobias include:

- acrophobia (fear of heights)
- aerophobia (fear of flying)
- apiphobia (fear of bees)
- arachnophobia (fear of spiders)
- claustrophobia (fear of confined spaces)
- dentophobia (fear of dentists)
- emetophobia (fear of vomiting)
- erythrophobia (fear of blushing)
- ophiophobia (fear of snakes)
- ornithophobia (fear of birds)
- trypanophobia (fear of injections).

Specific phobias can often be dealt with very easily by desensitisation (graduated exposure). They do not involve the fear of public humiliation or social failure as do the other groups of phobias and are therefore usually less complex to treat. Also, for example, the therapist can be with the child when trying to desensitise her to spiders; this is not always possible when the fear the child has involves a ride on a bus or speaking in class, although some therapists will accompany patients, for example, to school or on a bus journey.

Specific phobias also seem to be more easily understood by the majority as most people have at least one of these fears themselves; the type of fear is similar and is limited to one particular thing. When fears are more general, as with agoraphobia and social phobia, unless people have personally suffered something similar they find it hard to comprehend. To them, doing the things that frighten agoraphobics and social phobics is a part of normal everyday living. Even when someone close to them suffers from one of these conditions, they lack the same understanding, whether for a fellow child or as an adult trying to understand a child. This makes it harder for children and their parents to admit to needing help or in understanding the best way to help.

Panic attacks

A panic attack is an extreme response to an anxious event, usually starting following the onset of a phobia (at least initially; once a child starts having panic attacks it is possible to have them without any particular stimulus). The symptoms are very distressing and can include:

- abdominal pain

- chest pains or discomfort in the chest

- chills or feeling very hot

- choking

- feeling dizzy or faint (this can be brought on by hyperventilation because the mix of the gases in the blood changes, having too much oxygen and too little carbon dioxide); the child can actually faint

- frequent need to urinate (and the child may have diarrhoea)

- nausea and vomiting

- numbness or tingling feelings (from hyperventilating)

- palpitations

- quick shallow breathing (hyperventilation) is very common (the child feels she can't breathe and so over-breathes in panic)

- rapid heartbeat

- shaking

- shortness of breath

- suddenly feeling hot or cold

- sweating.

As well as experiencing the above symptoms (of which at least four need to be present for the event to be classed as a full panic attack), a child may have psychological symptoms. These could be:[3]

- derealisation (feeling that the world is not real; feeling detached from everything around)

- depersonalisation (feeling detached from her own body, feeling unreal and cut off from herself or losing her personal identity)

- feeling out of control

- feeling terrified

- feeling she will go mad

- feeling she might die.

The length of time a panic attack can last varies from a few minutes to several hours (particularly if the child remains in the environment that caused the panic attack).

It is little wonder that, once a child has experienced a panic attack, she is reluctant to leave the safety of her home, fearing another attack without the comforting presence of a parent.

Why do panic attacks start?

Panic attacks are usually preceded by some form of increased stress. They can start if a child is highly stressed for a long time and it is not relieved in some way, such as by resolving the situation that caused the stress, removing the cause of the stress or by dealing with it through exercise, having fun times to negate the stress and talking about it. Once a child is highly stressed, any further stress may push her past her personal threshold of stress tolerance, leading to a panic attack.

Sometimes, panic attacks are due to perceived fears rather than actual fears. An example of this is when a child has a phobia (or is starting to develop one). The negative thoughts that are generated in the child's mind when in a feared situation, or faced with something she is frightened of, create great anxiety. (Many of these thoughts may be sub-conscious as younger children are often unable to explain the thoughts they have that lead to a panic attack.) If the child is then unable to leave the situation or avoid the thing that frightens her, her negative thoughts escalate, feeding off the physical symptoms of her anxiety, proving to herself that she is right to be afraid. Very soon these panicky feelings can lead to a panic attack.

Some children are more prone to anxiety than others because of their personality. Personality type A people are more ambitious, very self-critical, perfectionist, prone to stress, impatient and cannot cope easily with changes in routine, whereas personality type B people are calmer, more relaxed, less prone to stress and take changes to routine in their stride. Children with personality type A will become panicky with a lower threshold of stress than those children with personality type B. Sometimes children have a combination of personality types with one usually predominating, but this is not always the case: they can be equally balanced.[4]

Children with *persistent* (beyond the expected years) behavioural inhibition (when a child is unusually shy or shows fear or withdrawal in *unfamiliar* situations) are more likely to suffer anxiety disorders such as panic disorder and social phobia than children without the trait. And children that have shown behavioural inhibition are more predisposed to anxiety generally, but do not necessarily develop an anxiety disorder.[5] Social shyness and inhibition are mostly passed on through the genes. It is believed that inhibited children are born with a nervous system that is more easily stressed and excited when faced with a novel social situation.[6]

Children are also more prone to anxiety if they have other family members who suffer from anxiety disorders (although anyone can suffer from them if the anxiety levels are high enough for long enough, individual thresholds for stress varying) or because of an environmental link: if children see their parents become anxious about everyday things they too can become anxious, believing that it is the normal way to react to such situations. Also, over-protective parenting can make a child more prone to anxiety as can heavy criticism and excessive punishment.[7]

Some children experience anxiety and have anxiety disorders as a result of a particular medical condition such as Asperger syndrome or high-functioning autism (the number of children being diagnosed with these conditions is increasing all the time). These children are particularly prone to bullying and social rejection (see *Anxiety: children with autistic spectrum disorders* below and *Refusing school: children with autistic spectrum disorders* in Chapter One; mention is also made in Chapter Three on *Bullying* and in Chapter Five on *Social phobia*). With a few children there is no apparent trigger for their anxiety.

Stressful life events can affect the child's mental health and make her more prone to anxiety disorders and panic attacks. Sometimes these life stresses are so intense that the child can suffer from post-traumatic stress disorder (see *Post-traumatic stress disorder* later in the chapter). Triggers can include serious illness, child abuse, witnessing a traumatic event or being part of one (a traumatic event being anything outside the normal everyday experience for that child) and bereavement.

Panic disorder

Panic disorder is diagnosed when children have unexpected and repeated periods of intense fear or discomfort or have panicky symptoms (these are all panic attacks) that can last minutes or hours. Because these panic attacks can happen anywhere at any time, the child worries about when the next one might be. Anxiety about having another panic attack can interfere with her life. The child can become anxious about being anywhere from where she cannot escape a situation should she feel panicky and may depend too much on her parents, feeling insecure when they are absent. The child may not want to go to school, feeling unsafe when she is away from home and her parents. And she might not feel safe with other adults looking after her, such as when going out with a friend and his parents.

The child's world can shrink with each panic attack. For example, if the child has a panic attack on a bus she might thereafter avoid travelling on buses. Then she might avoid going on trains too, and anywhere else that she feels panicky, fearing that it is the situations that cause the panic rather than her thinking patterns. With panic disorder, the anxiety is said to be 'free-floating' because it is not focused on a single event or situation and is therefore harder to treat than panic attacks associated with a particular trigger.

Panic disorder can begin in childhood but more commonly starts in adolescence. There is sometimes a link with another member of the same close family who suffers from panic attacks.

If the child's family doctor can find no physical cause for her symptoms, she should be referred to a child and adolescent mental health service. A child may be able to recognise panic attacks as isolated incidents when she has had counselling (if she is old enough to benefit from it), can learn to change the way she thinks about them and so never develop panic disorder, but there are no guarantees.

Untreated panic disorder may lead to agoraphobia (where a child does not want to travel on public transport or be anywhere where there is no means of immediate escape) and depression (because of the awful panicky feelings and the loss of social support that arises from not forming and maintaining close relationships). Other anxiety disorders can also coexist with panic disorder. Adolescents risk damping their fears through substance or alcohol abuse, failing or dropping out of school, or becoming socially isolated and almost housebound.[1] There is a risk that a child who has suffered panic disorder in childhood can be affected by it later on in life. A few never recover and may develop other psychiatric disorders and be socially impaired.

Panic disorder and separation anxiety

Panic disorder and separation anxiety (see Chapter Four) are closely linked. Either one can cause the other to develop if the child does not receive help, as mentioned above.

If a child develops panic attacks or panic disorder in childhood, she may well develop separation anxiety, never feeling safe when away from her parent, even in adulthood.

Separation anxiety in childhood can trigger panic disorder in adulthood. Children who do not develop (or who are discouraged from developing) independence in a secure environment may continue to feel anxious, without the support of a parent, into adulthood. When separation finally becomes inevitable (such as through the death of her parents), the person may not be able to cope.

Generalised anxiety disorder

A child who suffers from generalised anxiety disorder worries about everyday things far more than the situation or event warrants. The anxiety is low level and ever present. The child's anxiety is concentrated on things that are happening, or are about to happen, rather than worrying about the possibility of having a panic attack (as in panic disorder), or about not being able to cope travelling on the school bus (as in agoraphobia), or about being ill (as in hypochondria) or about going to school (as in school phobia). The anxiety is far more general and is considered to be 'free-floating' as in panic disorder. For a diagnosis of generalised anxiety disorder to be given, the child must have had excessive anxiety and worry for the majority of days over a six month period.[8] The child's anxiety should involve a number of situations, be hard to control and involve at least one of the following symptoms:

- being easily tired
- being irritable
- feeling restless
- finding it hard to concentrate
- finding it hard to get to sleep or to stay asleep
- having muscle tension.

Also, the anxiety or physical symptoms must cause significant distress or a reduction of normal day-to-day functioning.

With generalised anxiety disorder, the child's symptoms are similar to those of panic but are more persistent and less intense. It is thought that, as with panic disorder, generalised anxiety disorder is genetically linked in some cases, so that the sufferer inherits a predisposition to anxiety. A child suffering from generalised anxiety disorder may be seen to:

- avoid group activities such as after-school clubs and sports
- be a perfectionist
- be concerned about her performance and capabilities
- be overly anxious about her social behaviour and her social success
- be reluctant to, or refuse to, attend school
- be unable to relax
- be very self-conscious
- dislike being the centre of attention
- have difficulty speaking in group settings such as at school
- have nervous habits such as nail biting, hair pulling or foot or finger tapping
- have obsessive self-doubt
- have physical complaints not related to a specific situation, such as backache, stomachache, headaches or general malaise
- need constant reassurance
- ponder over the appropriateness of past behaviour
- want to excel academically, athletically and socially
- worry over what she is to wear the next day or how she looks
- worry too much about forthcoming events.

Obsessive compulsive disorder

Obsessions are inappropriate and dominating thoughts or images (not simply about being over-anxious about real-life problems) that recur in the child's head, causing her distress. The child tries to suppress or ignore these unwelcome thoughts or images and may recognise that the concerns are not real but are rooted in her own misguided mind, but is powerless to do anything about them.

Compulsions are repeated actions that are performed because of these thoughts or images; the child having to check and recheck that the action has been carried out properly or to perform certain tasks in a ritualistic way. If these behaviours are not carried out, the child's stress will mount. The behaviour is recognised by the child as being essential to put her mind at rest even though the need to do it is not grounded in reality.

A child's compulsion may involve repeated hand washing when she is particularly concerned about germs. She may not believe that the first time she washed her hands was adequate. She may have missed a bit or not used sufficient soap. Later she may touch something and believe that her hands have become contaminated again and that she will get sick if she does not wash them right away.

Other common compulsions in children are straightening (such as bed covers, cushions, curtains, towels), checking (that tasks have been carried out such as straightening correctly or tidying things in a certain way) and hoarding (being unable to throw anything away, including rubbish). Very often, checking has to be done in a certain order each time it is carried out and the child may have to perform special actions or repeat certain words each time a check has been made (when the compulsive behaviour includes rituals).

The child can spend several hours each day thinking about the obsessions and carrying out compulsive actions. She may be prevented from going to school because of her obsessive compulsive behaviour. For example, she may be very anxious about the state of her bedroom, feeling unable to leave her room until everything in it is tidy and in exactly the right place (and at the right angle). This may take her so long that she is made late for school. Sometimes a child can be anxious that someone might go in and disturb her room while she is out and so eventually cannot leave home at all. This is not a fear of the school environment but anxiety about leaving home, the child feeling she has to guard her room.

A child with obsessive compulsive disorder needs to be referred to a child and adolescent mental health service, as the condition tends to worsen with time.

Post-traumatic stress disorder

Some traumatic events that have caused post-traumatic stress disorder (PTSD) in children are: natural disasters such as earthquakes, cyclones and floods, and man-made disasters such as collapsed buildings and bombings; transport accidents such as car, coach, aeroplane or train crashes; violent crimes such as kidnapping, rape, murder or school shootings; severe burns; domestic or community violence such as racist attacks and gang wars; war; peer suicide; physical and sexual abuse; serious illnesses and bereavement. The child has either experienced the trauma personally or has witnessed it.

Children suffering from PTSD live in a constant state of fearfulness, reliving the experience over and over again in their play, their sleep, their drawings, their speech or their relationships with others. A child may be so badly affected by a distressing single event or by a chronic stressor (such as when a child is physically or sexually abused) that the anxiety she felt at the time is relived again and again. Some children have problems additional to PTSD including anxiety, depression, anger, aggression, low self-esteem and problems in their relationships.[9]

In order for a diagnosis of PTSD to be made (using ICD-10 classification), the onset of symptoms must follow a latency period, which may range from a few weeks to a few months (but rarely exceeds six months). If the onset of symptoms were immediate, they would give rise to a different diagnosis such as an adjustment disorder or acute stress reaction. The main symptoms of PTSD are:

1. The child is on edge all the time, waiting for something else bad to happen or for the same thing to happen again. The child may have difficulty falling or staying asleep, be irritable or have angry outbursts; have difficulty concentrating; be always on the alert (hypervigilance) or have an exaggerated startle response (such as jerking her body nervously in a very obvious way at the slightest unfamiliar sound).

2. The child has intrusive memories and nightmares as she repeatedly relives the experiences (termed 're-experiencing phenomena'). These reminders of the stressful event may be so strong that the child experiences a panic attack in a similar situation or becomes panicky at the mention of it or something similar. She may become very distressed if she is reminded of the traumatic event and may often feel as though she is reliving it. She may repeatedly enact the traumatic event through play.

3. The child has a feeling of unreality, in which she loses touch with normal life and her feelings (termed 'emotional numbness').

It is very common for a child suffering from post-traumatic stress disorder to have panic attacks and suffer from depression, and she is likely to persistently avoid anything that reminds her of the traumatic event. She may experience guilt (at not preventing the thing from happening or feeling that she was in some way to blame, or for surviving the experience when others didn't) and she may regress in her behaviour by acting younger than her age. She may also develop relationship problems with peers and family members, and have problems with school performance.

Factors that increase the likelihood of children developing post-traumatic stress disorder are:

- The severity and number of traumatic events. Personal traumas, such as rape and assault, are more likely to cause PTSD.

- The parental reaction to the traumatic event. Children who have a supportive family and whose parents cope well with the distress of the event have fewer and less severe post-traumatic stress symptoms.

- How close in time the child is to the traumatic event. The greater the distance, the less distress the child has.

If parents think the child is suffering from post-traumatic stress, they should seek help from a professional who specialises in PTSD, as the way it presents in children is age specific and can be different to how it affects adults. For example, a child might believe in omens and the prediction of disastrous future events, and have other problems additional to the symptoms of PTSD, only some of which are mentioned above.[9]

Depression

It is very distressing for a child to suffer from anxiety and panic attacks. The world may have suddenly become a very hostile place to her before she has even had a chance to understand it properly in a positive environment. A child who has anxiety disorders is at risk from developing depression either at the time or later in childhood or adolescence. She may see no way through and feel a deep unhappiness for a prolonged period of time. It is not something that she can snap out of. Suffering from anxiety and depression significantly increases the risks of suicide and attempted suicide.

With some children, their depression may be in response to a distressing life event such as their parents divorcing or one of them dying. Some common symptoms of depression in children are:

- being more irritable, angry, agitated or hostile than normal

- crying

- fatigue

- having headaches and stomachaches

- feeling useless

- feeling worthless

- lack of concentration or ability to make decisions

- lack of interest in things going on around her and enjoying things less than she used to

- lethargy and lack of motivation to do anything at all

- not being able to sleep or stay asleep all night or sleeping much more than normal

- poor appetite and weight loss (in some cases it can be weight gain)

- thinking of death or suicide a great deal.

If parents think the child is depressed they should seek help from her doctor.

Bedwetting (enuresis)

There can be many reasons for a child to wet her bed beyond the age of five. Sometimes it is due to slow development of bladder control, which is often hereditary. Rarely it indicates a kidney or bladder problem and can sometimes be related to a sleep disorder. Sometimes the child's bedwetting may be due to emotional problems or anxiety.[10]

If a child starts bedwetting after months or years of being dry at night, there is likely to be an emotional cause, resulting from fear or insecurity (although not always). For example, she may have moved home, changed school, had a new sibling, have parents who are separating or divorcing, or suffered bereavement. If she is anxious about going to school, one of the ways her anxiety manifests itself may be through bedwetting. (Some children also soil themselves due to having diarrhoea from anxiety, or if they have been traumatised, regressing because of the distress of the event.)

A child cannot help wetting the bed at night and she should not be reprimanded. If the child regularly wets her bed, parents could try:

- limiting her drink at bedtime

- making sure she goes to the toilet just before she settles down for the night

- waking her early, or when they go to bed, to go to the toilet

- praising her when she goes a night without wetting herself

- avoiding punishments or making her feel bad about herself.[10]

If these methods don't work, and there is no medical reason for the child's bedwetting, parents could ask for her to be referred to a child and adolescent mental health team (although not all offer help for enuresis any more as it is very low priority work compared to the other demands on their time), or to a local enuresis nurse.

Dealing with anxiety and panic

Children suffering from generalised anxiety disorder, agoraphobia and social phobia, and panic attacks need to be taught to relax (although this is not possible for very young children and may not be possible for children with autistic spectrum disorders: see below) and how to breathe without hyperventilating. (See Chapter Five: *Using relaxation techniques* and the suggested relaxation cassettes and CDs in the *Useful Resources* section.) This type of breathing is known as diaphragmatic breathing, where the chest hardly moves at all when inhaling, all the breath being used to push the diaphragm down, causing the abdomen to rise. This is a relaxed way of breathing that babies and animals do automatically. As people get older, they commonly become tense and change the way they breathe, particularly in stressful situations.

Anxious children also need to be reassured and given alternative, helpful thoughts to replace negative ones, and they need to have their fears listened to and discussed in a reasoned way, to see them in perspective and to recognise defective thinking. This is part of cognitive therapy, described in Chapter Seven. And they do not need surprises – such as having to leave home immediately or they'll miss the bus. A steady, informed approach is preferable where, for example, the child is told that she now has 15 minutes to make sure she has everything she needs and is appropriately clothed for outdoors. An ordered life helps make the anxious child feel more secure (this is particularly true for children who have an autistic spectrum disorder, as discussed below).

Working to improve the child's social skills to make her more socially confident and successful also helps to alleviate some of her fears (see Chapter Five).

Anxiety: children with autistic spectrum disorders

Children with autistic spectrum disorders often suffer from extreme anxiety and panic, agoraphobia, social phobia and other fears because of their condition (see *Refusing school: children with autistic spectrum disorders* in Chapter One). They are also very prone to depression and may have obsessive compulsive behaviour at a level to be classed as obsessive compulsive disorder. There are certain areas of these children's lives that they find difficult and respond to with anxiety.

ROUTINE

Children with autistic spectrum disorders often take comfort in routine (see also *Keep to the same routine* in Chapter Six) and can be anxious if it changes, being unable to predict what might happen next. They tend to meticulously plan for something by having either written or mental checklists.

The idea of routine for a child with an autistic spectrum disorder does not just mean to get up at the same time each day, have breakfast and go to school. It may mean to get up at 7.00, get dressed at 7.05 (the clothes selected and put out the night before: the child may want to wear the same clothes every day or be particular about what else he will wear), be downstairs at 7.20, eat breakfast (which may be the same food the child has for breakfast every morning without the slightest deviation) and so on. Any unexpected event that interferes with this routine can cause immense stress to the child.

If the child has a packed lunch at school, he may like to have a sandwich timetable (if what he's prepared to eat is sufficiently varied to allow for one) such as: Mondays: ham, Tuesdays: cheese and so on, which will help him with his need for order and repetitiveness.

As a reaction to stress and anxiety, a child with an autistic spectrum disorder will impose an even greater routine or ritual upon his life in order to cope with his distress.[11]

New situations provoke anxiety as these children are unable to be flexible or adaptable, so if a change is unavoidable the situation should be explained to the child and someone should stay with him throughout to support him and repeat the explanations of what will happen when. He needs to be prepared in advance for changes in routine such as sports day, assemblies, having a visiting speaker, days out, inset days (teaching staff's in-service training days) and exams.

Unstructured break times, or when the child has finished a task and there is nothing specific for him to do, may cause anxiety. Teachers could tell the child to read a particular magazine or book (it would be a problem to ask the child to choose a book when the choice itself could cause anxiety). (The child could come to school prepared for such times and have something in his bag to occupy him.)

CHANGING ACTIVITY

Children with autistic spectrum disorders may need time between activities to adjust to what is to come. For example, when it is break time the other children in the class will instantly get up and get what they need for their break, but a child with an autistic spectrum disorder will need time to think about what he needs to do and to understand the difference between directed and non-directed time, and will need time to adapt. Switching from one activity to another in a hurry might not be possible for the child and could cause him anxiety. He may need to be told what will happen next and what is expected of him.

SEQUENCING OF EVENTS

A child with an autistic spectrum disorder may have problems in sequencing events and so may need a chart (or cards with an activity on each one, placed on a board in a certain order) to let him know the order of things he needs to do. If the order has to be changed for some reason this should be explained to the child and the chart (or order of the cards) will also need to change, as the child is likely to check and recheck what he is meant to be doing.

For example, the child may struggle to be punctual: he may need much time to get ready to go to school and may need clear instructions of the stages involved. He may also need to be constantly reminded of them. (Parents could have a chart in his bedroom that the child can consult showing the time he gets out of bed, the time he must go downstairs, the time he must start his breakfast, when he must be finished by, when he cleans his teeth, gets dressed, goes downstairs again, etc.) Being given the sequence one day does not mean the child will be able to remember it on a subsequent day or adapt it to suit another occasion.

DECISION-MAKING

Children with autistic spectrum disorders can experience anxiety when presented with choice. Such a child is often unable to make decisions: the more choices available to him, the greater his level of anxiety. Parents can help the child in his decision-making either by making the decision for him or by gradually exposing him to a decision-making environment.

For example, they could slowly introduce the element of choice by initially giving only two alternatives: 'Would you like chicken or ham for dinner?' or 'Would you like to wear this T-shirt or that one?' Even in a full menu or full set of clothes there can be too much choice initially. Also, the child may have no idea, for example, which clothes are suitable for what weather or activity or if they match. Too many variables distress the child.

SOCIAL SITUATIONS

Children with autistic spectrum disorders find all social contact stressful, as they cannot process nonverbal (body language) information as other children can. They find it hard both to interpret any meaning that is not literal (see *Refusing school: children with autistic spectrum disorders* in Chapter One) and to give appropriate responses. Being teased or ridiculed over something the child cannot understand can distress him and he may eventually develop social phobia.

Dealing with anxiety in children with autistic spectrum disorders

This section considers the best way to help children with autistic spectrum disorders overcome anxieties during the day (helping such children get to sleep is looked at in *Routine to help sleep* in Chapter Six). (Also see *Using relaxation techniques* in Chapter Five.)

Children with autistic spectrum disorders can become very tired through having high levels of anxiety and by having to work so hard at trying to process all the social information given to them and cope with their co-ordination (see *Refusing school: children with autistic spectrum disorders* in Chapter One). Consequently, they may need to take a break.

In school a child with an autistic spectrum disorder will benefit from breaks when his anxiety starts to mount. He could be allowed to sit in a quiet corner of the class or the school library, where he could read, do a crossword puzzle (at home he could listen to relaxing music) or become immersed in his special interest (these are common among children with autistic spectrum disorders), or he could spend time on the computer. These things help to relax him through distraction, change of pace and time out.

Going on an errand, if he likes to do that sort of thing, may help through the small amount of exercise he will get when walking and because of having a break in the activity he was doing at the time. (Some children respond to having exercise when anxious, so could be given things to do around the house or school or be taken out for physical play.) Some children may need regular breaks such as this and, if so, instead of waiting for the child to show a need for them, it would help if his needs were anticipated by timetabling them into his personal home and school schedule.

If the child's anxiety is generally very high he may need a longer break than those just described. (This will probably be evident from his coping behaviours: becoming more rigid in his routine and retreating into his special interest with more avidity than usual.) This might mean he has a few days off school to unwind and regain his emotional balance, attend part-time or even be educated at home for a while.[12] (Also see *Special schools for children with autistic spectrum disorders* in Chapter One.) If the child is upset or anxious, it may be inappropriate to offer physical comfort or verbal reassurance as this can increase the child's irritation and anxiety. What he needs is space, with the knowledge that there is understanding and help when needed.[13]

As all children are individual, cautious trial and error will help identify which methods suit, what to do when and which methods to avoid. And most of all, attention should be paid to what the child says he needs or shows he needs, rather than what adults think he needs. Independence should not be forced on the child if he is not ready for it, regardless of what other children his age are doing, and adults should accept the child's coping mechanisms (such as a very rigid routine and immersion in his special interest).

Conclusion

Any number of things can trigger anxiety in a child and very often it is hard to distinguish whether her symptoms are from a physical illness or from anxiety. Parents know the child best and are therefore the best judge of whether persistent unspecific symptoms are from an illness or worry, and may well instinctively know to tread carefully if they think the child is under stress. (If in doubt, they could have the child checked by her doctor; there may be an underlying physical cause to the child's symptoms.)

Finding out the cause of the child's stress may be no easy task. Younger children particularly have difficulty in expressing themselves and may not even be aware of what it is that upsets them. They just know they don't want to go somewhere or do something but cannot verbalise the reasons why. So it is up to parents to try to play detective. If they are convinced that something is troubling the child, they should involve her class teachers and ask for their help.

Anxiety is a limiting illness, preventing children from living happy, carefree and outgoing lives. It is therefore important to take any child's anxieties seriously, no matter how ridiculous they seem, and work at ways to relieve them. If the child regularly experiences a parent's immediate attention regarding an anxiety, and has the situation explained to her to reduce or take away her fear, she will be more likely to accept that the world is not such a frightening place. And worrying thoughts are then less likely to spiral in her head, unbeknown to the parent, magnifying the importance of her fears and causing unpleasant anxiety symptoms.

References

1.   www.klis.com/chandler/pamphlet/panic/part2.htm

2.   www.familymedicine.co.uk/novarticles/socphobia.htm

3.   National Phobics Society factsheet *Panic Attacks/Panic Disorder* (see *Useful Contacts*).

4.   Kirsta, A. (1986) *The Books of Stress Survival: How to Relax and Live Positively.* London: Gaia Books, p.24.

5.   www.mcmaster.ca/inabis98/ameringen/coplan0344/index.html

6.   www.healthyplace.com/communities/anxiety/anxieties/3social/intro1.htm

7.   www.mcevoy.demon.co.uk/medicine/psychiatry/childpsych/anxphobs/predisps.html

8.   www.anxietycare.org.uk/documents/separation%20anxiety.htm

9.   www.psychcentral.com/library/ptsd_child.htm

10. www.aacap.org/publications/factsfam/bedwet.htm

11. Attwood, T. (1998) *Asperger's Syndrome*. London: Jessica Kingsley Publishers, p.100.

12. Ibid. p.156.

13. puterakembara.org/aspie.shtml

Further reading

Web addresses for further information and advice on anxiety disorders:

www.phobialist.com (This website lists phobias.)

www.aacap.org/publications/factsfam/noschool.htm (Webpages on separation anxiety.)

www.childpsychotherapists.com/sepanxiety.html (Webpages on separation anxiety.)

www.apa.org/practice/traumaticstress.html (Webpages on PTSD from the American Psychological Association.)

www.aacap.org/publications/factsfam/ptsd70.htm (Webpages on PTSD from the American Academy of Child and Adolescent Psychiatry.)

www.childtrauma.com/chpinf.html (Webpages on PTSD.)

mentalhelp.net/disorders/sx28.htm (Webpages on panic disorder.)

www.nmha.org/children/children_mh_matters/depression.cfm (Webpages on depression in children.)

www.aacap.org/publications/factsfam/depressed.htm (Webpages on depression in children from the American Academy of Child and Adolescent Psychiatry.)

www.rcpsych.ac.uk (The Royal College of Psychiatrists website.)

www.adaa.org (Anxiety Disorders Association of America website.)

www.mentalhealth.com/fr00.html (Internet Mental Health website.)

www.phobics-society.org.uk (National Phobics Society.)

Information and advice on high-functioning autism and Asperger syndrome can be found at the following web addresses:

www.nas.org.uk/pubs/asd/index.html (The National Autistic Society website. Contains information and advice on autism and Asperger syndrome.)

www.autism-society.org (Website of the Autism Society of America containing information on autism.)

www.udel.edu/bkirby/asperger/oasis (Online Asperger syndrome Information and Support.)

www.aspie.org (Asperger's Syndrome Parent Information Environment website.)

www.angelfire.com/amiga/aut (A personal website describing Asperger syndrome.)

www.vaporia.com/autism/ (Information and links on autism and Asperger syndrome.)

Books

Curtis, J. (2002) *Does Your Child Have a Hidden Disability?* London: Hodder & Stoughton.
This book was written for the large number of parents who find themselves worrying about whether there is something not quite right with their child, and finding it difficult to pinpoint just what is wrong and where to look for help. 'Invisible' disabilities are among the most distressing of all childhood problems, the most common being: attention deficit disorder, auditory attention problems, Asperger syndrome, autism, dyslexia, asthma, depression, allergies, learning difficulties and speech and language problems. It is not a medical book but instead focuses on the social and emotional impact of these disabilities on the whole family.

Moyes, R.A. (2001) *Incorporating Social Goals in the Classroom.* London: Jessica Kingsley Publishers.
This book provides practical strategies to teach social skills to children with high-functioning autism and Asperger syndrome and is suitable for use by parents and teachers.

Graham, P. and Hughes, C. (1995) *So Young, So Sad, So Listen.* London:
    Gaskell Publications.
This book was written in collaboration with the Royal College of Psychiatrists
and is concerned with depression in children and young people. Although the
book is intended mainly for parents and teachers, it could also be of interest to
professionals and teenagers.

Munden, A. and Arcelus, J. (1999) *The AD/HD Handbook: A Guide for
    Parents and Professionals on Attention Deficit/Hyperactivity Disorder.* London:
    Jessica Kingsley Publishers.
This book provides a comprehensive account of current knowledge of ADHD
and offers practical advice to parents, teachers, social workers and other professionals working with young people and their families.

World Health Organization (WHO) (1992) *The ICD-10 Classification of
    Mental and Behavioural Disorders.* Geneva: World Health Organization.

Factsheets

Mental Health and Growing Up: Factsheets for Parents, Teachers and Young People.
    (1999) London: Gaskell Publications. Published by the Royal College
    of Psychiatrists (see *Useful Contacts*).

Chapter Three

Bullying

Being aware of any kind of bullying behaviour will help the child identify such behaviour, deal with it in a positive way and, if the child is likely to have regular contact with the 'bullying' child, help her to protect herself.

What is bullying?

Bullying is singling out a child (it is rarely a couple or group of people) for victimisation or negative treatment that is repeated over a period of time. It involves an unfair balance of power, which makes it hard for the bullied child to defend herself.

A child cannot be thought of as bullied for a single event, even though she may have been at the brunt of bullying behaviour. Although this is unpleasant and can hurt a child, it is not as serious as systematically destroying a child's self-esteem or deliberately isolating her from friends.

Bullying can be direct, where there is open hostility for anyone to observe if they are present, or indirect, which is subtler, a teacher often failing to observe it or recognise it as bullying. Overall, most bullying is done by boys and they are most likely to use physical means on other boys, but indirect methods on girls. Most bullying done by girls is indirect.[1] However, Rigby suggests that the trend for girls and women is changing to that of being more aggressive, violent and more inclined to bully, as women feel the need to show that they too are tough and not 'wimps'.[2]

Direct bullying can include:

- Deliberately tripping up a child so that she is hurt or made to look ridiculous.

- Physically hurting a child (kicking, punching, scratching, hair pulling).

- Restraining a child or preventing her from leaving a room (such as the school toilets). This could be to make the child late for class or to miss a bus home or simply to frighten her.

- Threatening to harm a child or forcing her to do something under threat of some kind.

Indirect bullying can include:

- Name-calling and taunting.

- Making threatening faces or gestures at a child or using rude body language to demean the child, such as nose-holding when a particular child walks into the room.

- Pretending to befriend a child and then telling everyone her secrets or fears.

- Prolonged unkind teasing. (For example, making fun of the way someone speaks, dresses or is different in some way, by reason of her race, sexuality or disability.)

- Provocative behaviour (such as wearing racist badges or insignia).

- Sending nasty emails.

- Splitting up friendships and isolating a child so that she has no one to play with.

- Spreading gossip or rumours.

- Stealing a child's best friend so that she will be on her own.

- Taking or hiding another child's possessions.

- Texting nasty mobile 'phone messages.

Who are the bullies?

Bullies are people who have power over others who are seemingly weaker or disadvantaged in some way due to lack of confidence, shyness or disability. This might be because of a superior position (such as being an older child or being more experienced than the bullied child), or because of greater strength or popularity.

Bullies often have a problem with their home life or upbringing that they cannot cope with, such as home stresses that they suffer personally, or see happen to another family member. These include unemployment, divorce, alcoholism, bereavement, imprisonment and violence.

A bully is someone who:

- likes to have power over others

- likes to make others do things she asks

- likes to frighten people

- likes to humiliate people

- likes to get her own way

- is probably bullied at home or lives with an aggressive parent

- needs help.

Why children bully

Bullies may:

- Have experienced ineffectual parenting where threats of punishment are not carried through, effectively rewarding them for negative behaviour. (Only when their parents are sufficiently riled is action taken and then it may be violent and extreme.)

- Be modelling behaviour that their parents use towards them.

- Want to have their own way, at any cost, and do not care who this might hurt.

- Have feelings that are not understood and needs that are not addressed, making them feel bitter and angry, and so they take out their frustration on someone they see as weaker than themselves. Or the bullies might be victims of abuse and take out their hurt on others.

- Have not had a positive role model and so do not know how to handle feelings of anger and frustration without resorting to violence or manipulation (social threats).

- Not have high self-esteem and so need to prove themselves stronger than others and need to feel in control, by getting others to do what they want.

- Act aggressively to attract attention, feeling negative attention is better than none.

- Have become involved with others who display anti-social behaviour and copy theirs to be in with the group or gang.

- Be jealous of others who are richer, have more friends or greater talent than themselves.

Why children become victims of bullying

Reasons why children can become victims of bullying:

- They are just unlucky to be in the wrong place at the wrong time.

- They display passive or timid body language so bullies identify them as likely targets.

- They have little confidence so are not good at standing up for themselves.

- They are bullied at home and so accept their role as the downtrodden.

- They are perceived as being 'weak' in some way, such as not being good at sports.

- They do not wear the 'right' clothes (unfashionable clothes or non-designer trainers).

- They are different to the majority in some way: the way they look (such as having freckles, being very thin or fat, having an unfashionable hairstyle); their ethnic origin; the way they speak or because they have some disability (such as needing to wear glasses or a hearing aid, limping, having a speech impediment, having social impairments because of a medical condition such as an autistic spectrum disorder, or using a wheelchair).

- Their parents are different in some way to the majority, such as being over-protective, dressing unusually, having a different accent or being viewed as eccentric in some way.

- Their parents or other family members have particular problems or lifestyles that are known, such as alcoholism, drug addiction, imprisonment or multiple partners.

- They like attention, so create a big fuss about small things and get noticed by people who are eager to take advantage of them.

- They are seen as 'swots' or have a special talent that is not accepted by the majority (for example, a boy being good at dancing instead of the stereotypically acceptable football or rugby).

The effects bullying can have

Bullied children may:

- Remain socially passive, only speaking to those who speak to them first, never taking the initiative and not being the first to try to make a new friend.

- Be easily intimidated.

- Feel unable to cope.

- Be very lonely, being rejected by their peers.

- Become self-critical and self-hating, having a very low self-esteem.

- Become depressed and try to harm themselves.

(Also see *Bullying and physical and mental health* below.)

Are some children programmed for life to be bullied?

Some children seem to be programmed for life to be bullied. They are abused at home, which lowers their self-esteem; they are then bullied at school, further reducing their self-esteem; and they may end up in an abusing relationship. It is as though they have accepted this as their lot. (For some people it can take years of violence and abuse within a partnership before the person leaves for good, if ever.)

One bad experience of being bullied can change children, making them vulnerable to bullying in the future. Being bullied dents their confidence to the extent that their body language shows them to be timid people who can be taken advantage of. Bosses in the workplace often do bully or harass employees under their supervision.

Some children are bullied by chance. They are not abused at home, are confident and display confident body language, but something about them catches the fancy of the bully; it may be a passing whim. So the bullied child might not ever be bullied again.

What the child can do to protect herself from bullies

The child can:

- Try to avoid the bully whenever possible.

- Inform the bully when confronted and threatened that she will tell on him or her if she is not left alone. She must mean it and carry it through if necessary. She could tell her teacher, her parents or the police (if she's been physically hurt or has been seriously threatened).

- Try to avoid lonely places. For example, she shouldn't go to the toilets on her own if she feels unsafe or suspects the bully might be waiting there for her.

- Try to get witnesses to anything that has happened to her at the bully's hands to make people take her complaints seriously.

- Keep a diary of events detailing who said or did what, and when and where. This helps to build up evidence, particularly when there is no physical evidence of torn clothes and bruises. Much of bullying is insidious and hard to detect, so that complaints to teachers are not always taken seriously.

- Think up comments to say in reply if the bullying is verbal and not too threatening. She might be able to think up something that turns the put-down back on to the bully, making him or her feel silly. If she doesn't know what to say, she could ask the bully to repeat what he or she has just said as this might dent the person's confidence.

- Try not to let the bully know he or she has got to her; that takes away the satisfaction of bullying her. If she's not fun to bully, she might be left alone.

- Try to increase her confidence by becoming physically fit, learning to be assertive and learning confident body language (see Chapter Five). She should practise behaving in a confident way.

- Learn social skills (see Chapter Five) so that she is less likely to be a target in the future. Being able to appropriately express herself will get people to take her seriously, and being more socially skilled will help her to build strong friendships that can protect her from bullies who see isolated children as easy targets.

Why it is important to stop bullies
If bullies aren't stopped:

- They might go on to do worse things because they know they can get away with it.

- They can become more dangerous and can ruin their victims' lives.

- Other people might be encouraged to become bullies if they see others get away with it.

- They can potentially ruin another person's life. Some adults have needed counselling because of the effect bullying has had on them; it is not something the victim easily gets over – the memory and the feelings can remain with the person.

- They may, as adults, behave abusively to their partner and children. Many children who bully have been brought up in an abusive household, so they have had negative role models of parents, which they use to model their own behaviour.

Why bullies need help

Bullies should seek help as they could have happier and more fulfilling lives without the aggression and hate that builds up inside them. (Bullying also affects their physical and mental health: see below.) It might also stop them from going one step too far with their aggression and badly hurting or killing someone. If bullying behaviour is allowed to continue, the bullies' anti-social behaviour may lead to crime, spouse and child abuse, substance abuse and being only able to socialise with those who have similar behaviour, having alienated themselves from most others.

Bullying and physical and mental health

Many studies have shown that there is now a well established link between poor physical and mental health and bullying in schools, some of which are mentioned here. Rigby and Slee (1993)[3] found that bullied children were more likely to be unhappy than non-bullied children and that the contrasts were stronger for children under 13: frequently victimised girls under 13 were more than seven times as likely to see themselves as unhappy, and frequently victimised boys under 13 were more than three times as likely to see themselves as unhappy as non-bullied children.

Another study by Rigby and Slee (1993)[4] showed that bullies are significantly less happy than children who aren't victims or bullies, and that being victimised by peers significantly lowers self-esteem. Several studies have also found that frequently victimised children are significantly more depressed than others[5] and a Finnish study (1999)[6] showed that suicidal thoughts were significantly related to peer victimisation. Bullies too have higher than average thoughts about suicide (Rigby and Slee 1999).[7]

Olweus (1978)[8] reported that peer victimisation by aggressive peers can lead to chronic anxiety, and children aggressively bullied were significantly more anxious and insecure than others. Aggressive children followed to adulthood had increased risks of unemployment, criminal behaviour, spouse abuse, alcoholism, anti-social personality disorder and depression and anxiety.[9]

A study by Salmon et al. (1998)[10] also found that bullied children are more anxious than their peers, and bullies were found to have higher depression scores than those of their peers. Although children involved in bullying issues are mostly either bullies or victims, approximately 20 per cent of victims also act as bullies (bully/victims).[8]

Several studies have shown that children repeatedly victimised at school are lonelier, have an aversion to the school environment and are more likely to be absent from school than non-victimised children, and that absenteeism increases in relation to the severity of peer victimisation.[5] And Rigby and Slee (1993)[4] found that bullies do not like school as much as others do and are absent from school more often than most children, but this may be for different reasons to the bullied children as bullies may feel bored, seeking distractions outside school.

In a study by Salmon et al. (2000)[11] it was found that over 70 per cent of bullied adolescents referred to outpatient psychiatric services were diagnosed with depression compared to the control group, and half of the depressed bullied adolescents also had a history of deliberate self-harm, whereas bullies and bully/victims were most likely to present with conduct disorders that may coexist with ADHD.

There are longer term effects on social adjustment as found in a study by Tritt and Duncan (1997)[12] where American undergraduates aged 18 to 22 years who had been victimised at school were found to feel significantly more lonely than others. Another study in Australia by

Dietz (1994)[13] assessed the psychological well-being of both men and women who were victimised in school and found that they had marked difficulties in forming close intimate relationships with members of the opposite sex. Another study conducted in Scandinavia by Olweus (1992)[14] found that men in their early twenties who had been victimised in school, compared with other men, had significantly lower self-esteem, suggesting that peer victimisation can have enduring effects.[5]

Williams *et al.* (1996)[15] found that peer victimised primary school children were more than twice as likely as non-victimised children to say they had headaches and stomachaches. Other health symptoms due to peer victimisation may involve feeling sad or very sad, bedwetting and sleeping difficulties, so for children presenting with these symptoms, health professionals should consider bullying as a contributory factor.

Rigby (1998)[16] found that bullies are generally physically less well than other children and that boy bullies were more likely to report frequent vomiting, whereas girl bullies were more likely to report frequent mouth sores.

In an anonymous survey of Australian secondary school children by Rigby (1999),[17] bullied children had reported a higher incidence of emotional distress in the form of physical symptoms, anxiety, social dysfunction and depression, and more perceived adverse health effects such as headaches and mouth sores. Male bullies also consistently reported poorer health.

A study of Australian secondary school children by Forero *et al.* (1999)[18] found that bullying behaviour was associated with an increased number of psychosomatic symptoms (physical disorders that seem to have been caused or worsened by psychological factors such as headache, stomachache, backache, feeling low or irritable or in a bad temper, feeling nervous, difficulty in getting to sleep, feeling dizzy), psychological symptoms (such as loneliness, unhappiness, lack of confidence) and smoking, with those students who both bullied and were bullied reporting the highest frequency of symptoms. Bullies tended to be unhappy with school and students who were bullied tended to like school more but to report feeling alone (due to having few friends, being introverted and generally lacking social skills). Students who were bully/victims exhibited the characteristics of disliking school and feeling alone, and they seemed to have the most psychological and psychosomatic symptoms.

In conclusion, bullies, victims and bully/victims have poorer mental and physical health than other children and bully/victims are at highest risk from health problems. Consequently, health professionals should consider bullying and the child's school environment as potential causes of common psychological and psychosomatic symptoms.

Why does being bullied induce poor health?

Rigby[5] suggests frequent bullying can wear a child's personal resources to their limit and beyond, soon reaching a point where the child feels unable to cope. And the unpredictability of the attacks means that the child has little or no control over when something happens and no time to prepare for it. Sometimes the bully may ignore the child, at other times react in a hostile way and at others be charming, so that the child is confused. This adds another element of unpredictability. And the child's failure to cope can humiliate her and reduce her sense of self-worth, increasing the risk of suicidal thoughts.

Although the child may try different things to escape the bully or to get help, if these fail she is considerably more out of control of the situation. The child may also become more isolated and lonely. Severe stress in a child can lead to a range of health problems (as discussed above).

Why does bullying induce poor health?

Rigby[5] suggests that bullies' poor health may come from the home environment (such as being part of a dysfunctional family and having cold, over-controlling parents – things that are a factor in the rearing of bullies). Tendencies towards depression and suicidal thinking in bullies may be due to unskilful parenting and an unhappy home life that makes them miserable enough to want to take out their negative feelings on others.

How do adults know if the child is being bullied?

Children often try to hide the fact they are being bullied because they are scared of retaliation, scared that they will be thought of as a wimp or disbelieved by whomever they tell. Bullies can force the child not to talk or the child may feel that she needs to deal with it herself and that there is no other way.

As well as talking to the child, adults can observe her and see if they notice anything different about the way she behaves. Behavioural changes and other clues to look out for include the following:

- Is the child suddenly scared to walk to school, or come home from school, alone?

- Does she want to avoid any children from her school that she previously didn't mind being with?

- Does the child stay unusually close when out with her parents or when she sees any particular child or group of children?

- Does she have any marks on her body?

- Do her belongings mysteriously disappear?

- Do her belongings come home damaged, for which she can offer no explanation?

- Are her clothes splattered with mud? (This may indicate she has been pulled to the floor.)

- Does she ask for more money, saying she has lost her dinner money? (This could indicate extortion.)

- Have parents caught her stealing money from them? (This could also indicate extortion.)

- Does the child say negative things about herself such as 'I'm stupid' or 'I'm clumsy'? Does she use negative words about herself that have not been used to her at home? If so, who called her these names and why?

- Has she asked what something means, either a word or a sign, such as sticking two fingers in the air in a 'V' shape? (This could indicate the sign has been used to her.)

It is very important to ask the child about her day and her friendships to find out if she is being treated negatively. Even if she does not herself recognise the behaviour as bullying, adults would be able to identify it as such and talk it through with her, explaining why it is unreasonable. Ways for the child to deal with it could then be suggested.

A child should never be made to feel bad for having given 'inside' or 'privileged' information, because then she will stop telling. Instead of adults showing the child they are angry she didn't stand up for herself or that they're very angry at something a friend has done, they should ask her how she felt and whether she thought what happened was fair. Things she could do or say could be suggested or she could be asked to suggest solutions. The problem should be followed up by asking the child if it's happened again and if so, what did she do?

If she has tried to tackle the situation she should be praised, because it is important she looks after herself – no one has a right to make her feel bad when she has done nothing wrong.

Adults should show they are interested in things that happen to the child and talk openly about bullying behaviour not being nice, explaining that it will continue unless children speak out. Upon hearing this, the child is more likely to keep teachers and parents informed.

Some bullying can't be dealt with by the child. If the child is a boy, parents should not show disappointment that he 'can't stand up for himself and be a man' as that will destroy his self-esteem. It is up to parents to protect children, whatever their age and sex, and intervene by involving the school and the police if necessary. It may not be advisable to go directly to the parents of the bullying child unless it is certain that they will be sympathetic rather than denying that their child is at fault, which would only make matters worse. Using a third party such as the headteacher to intervene on parents' behalf will make them take the matter more seriously. This may bring to light other complaints about the same child that those parents would find even harder to ignore.

Suggestions to help a child who is excluded from a group of friends

If a group is refusing to let the child play with them when she has done so previously, talk to her to find out who the leader is. Who speaks up first and says 'No, she can't join in'? Who tells the others what to do? Parents could try to improve the bonds between the child and the *other* members of the group by inviting them to play with the child, and parents could discuss the problem with the class teacher. Teachers could try to get the other members of the group to work co-operatively with the child on class assignments. They might then stand up to the leader in support of the child. If this doesn't work, the teacher could tell the parents of the unkind children that their children are helping to exclude the child from the group.

In any case, parents and teachers should encourage the child to make as many friends as possible within the class. Parents can help by asking the child to choose one or two others whom she likes but has not played with much, and invite them home. Teachers can help by pairing her with another child who is likely to be receptive to making friends. Giving the child more friendship opportunities makes the leader/bully lose power. When it becomes no longer important for the child to play in that group, because she has made other friends, the group members may lose interest and stop excluding her from their games.

As primary school children get older their interests change. They may choose to play with children that like running around rather than staying with the friends they sit with, for example. Being prepared to play or socialise with different groups of children will increase their circle of social contact and will make them more secure, in that they don't rely on just one or two children for all their entertainment. It also makes them more confident and enables them to make their own decisions.

At secondary school, children may prefer to be recognised as being part of a particular group and be happy to get all their security, support and entertainment from this group, desperate to fit in and to be seen to fit in. Groups of older children often have much more in common, such as the music they like and the clothes they wear, and want to be clearly identified as being together and so may alter their dress (despite wearing a school uniform) to show this. For example, wearing a tie at a particular angle or degree of loosening, wearing knee socks that have been rolled or pushed down, wearing jumpers around their waists, or carrying their blazers over their shoulders.

At this age it is vital for children to feel that they fit in. Not fitting in can cause great anxiety and can make them feel socially awkward or excluded (see Chapter Five), making them a target for bullying and social rejection.

Bullying: children with autistic spectrum disorders

Children who have an autistic spectrum disorder are particularly prone to bullying and do not understand why their peers (and sometimes their teachers) are so unkind. They often have problems with motor skills, being clumsy and unco-ordinated (see *Refusing school: children with autistic spectrum disorders* in Chapter One), and stand out from others in not being able to socially relate to them or understand jokes and teasing.

The National Autistic Society[19] advises parents to ask the child's teacher if he or she could arrange to find a 'buddy' for him: an older child or a classmate who will look out for him and help him to join games in the schoolyard. Parents could also discuss the possibility of having a 'circle of friends' for the child, who will help integrate him into his peer group, so that he fits in better and is less open to bullying.

It should also be made clear to the child, if he is bullied, where he should go for help and whom to talk to. A child who is very upset and can't talk because of his stress may not be able to verbalise how he feels or what is wrong. If a chart showing faces with different expressions is available, he could point to the particular expression that explains how he feels. (He may first have to be taught to recognise the expressions as being related to particular feelings, as this is nonverbal feedback which such children can have difficulty recognising.)

Bullying prevention

Forero *et al.* (1999)[18] recommend a positive school environment that does not tolerate bullying, engaging the help of children not involved in bullying to reduce the tolerance of bullying and change attitudes towards it. Schools should have a strong anti-bullying policy and pupils should be told that if they give information about bullying they need not worry that others will find out.

Teachers need to take heed of what their pupils say and act on any information that indicates bullying. A bully may test the teacher to see what his or her boundaries of acceptable behaviour are. For example, if a bully displays minor threatening behaviour towards another child, how the teacher reacts to witnessing this or being told about it may affect that bully's behaviour in the future. If the teacher is seen to take the matter seriously, the bully may not try again. But if the teacher ignores it or does not show concern for the victim, the bully will know that he or she can get away with more.

Similarly, if the bully tests the victim on a small matter and the victim does not complain to an adult such as a teacher, the bully may feel encouraged to go further. Victims need to show they recognise bullying behaviour and are not prepared to tolerate it.

Teachers can also take the trouble to notice if a pupil has been crying or looks sad, and ask what is wrong when they are alone together. (A victim may brush off any troubles if publicly asked what the problem is.) Teachers overtly showing a caring attitude towards their pupils will encourage pupils to offer confidences about matters that cause them concern.

To help address the problem of aggressive boys, senior male pupils and male teachers should take a proactive role in stopping bullying behaviour, show expectations of positive social behaviour and show by their own behaviour in class and in dealing with others that they do not use aggression themselves.

The help of peers is essential as they are often present when bullying is going on, and so can directly intervene on the victim's behalf. However, they need to be taught to intervene appropriately. Just watching the bullying without intervening reinforces the act. Peers who show approval of the bully's behaviour will only encourage further bullying. If their approval is withdrawn, the bully will not get the desired attention and approval from them and so will not be encouraged to keep doing it. They also need to be aware that a victim who is socially isolated and withdrawn may not be able to tell anyone about what is happening, so peers can take on that responsibility themselves. Bullying is a whole school issue where parents, teachers and pupils should all work together for the common aim of having a safe and caring environment in which to learn.

Some schools train senior pupils, representatives from each year or volunteers from any year as peer support who are available at break times in a designated room for other pupils to go to for advice and support on a range of issues. Childline in Partnership with Schools (CHIPS) runs schemes to train pupils in peer support and can tailor the training to individual schools' needs, including helping both bullies and the bullied (details at the end of the chapter). Senior pupils such as sixth-formers or prefects could be specially trained to look for bullying behaviour and report it, and to support victims.

Bullying and positive behaviour can be included in the curriculum. It might be an important part of personal social and health education (my book, *Contentious Issues: Discussion Stories for Young People*, has several stories covering issues of bullying, intimidation and sexual and racial harassment for 11 to 18 year olds) or it could be brought up as a special issue.

Parents can help prevent their children being bullied by teaching them social and assertiveness skills, helping them to develop high self-esteem (see Chapter Five and my book, *Social Awareness Skills for Children*) and showing them how to behave responsibly and caringly towards others. They should also impress upon the child that no one has a right to negatively affect her life and so any bullying behaviour must be stopped, by getting adult help and the support of friends.

Parents can help their children not become bullies by teaching positive social behaviour and respect for others, and by not being over-strict, violent or aggressive towards them or allowing them to witness aggressive or violent behaviour between themselves.

Conclusion

Bullying that is not effectively and quickly sorted out can make a child's life a misery. Adults should listen to the child and not let any comment of hers that relates to bullying pass by, even if it is about bullying of other children in the school. They should find out what has happened, discuss the bullies' behaviour and insist the child always tells an adult about anything, no matter how small, that upsets her.

Without help, bullies may see no reason to change their behaviour, particularly if they find it gets them what they want. Small bullies can then grow into big bullies and become much harder to deal with (and much more dangerous). Therefore it is kinder to both bully and victim in the long run to tell all and get it stopped.

Remember, no one has a right to negatively affect the child's life for his or her own amusement.

References

1. Olweus, D. (1993) *Bullying at School.* Oxford: Blackwell Publishing, pp.18–19.

2. Rigby, K. (2002) *New Perspectives on Bullying.* London: Jessica Kingsley Publishers, p.180.

3. Rigby, K. and Slee, P.T. (1993) *The Peer Relations Questionnaire (PRQ).* Adelaide: University of South Australia.

4. Rigby, K. and Slee, P.T. (1993) 'Dimensions of interpersonal relating among Australian school children and their implications for psychological well-being'. *Journal of Social Psychology 133,* 1, 33–42.

5. Rigby, K. (2002) *New Perspectives on Bullying.* London: Jessica Kingsley Publishers, Chapter 5.

6. Kaltiala-Heino, R., Rimpela, M., Marttunen, M., Rimpela, A. and Rantanen, P. (1999) 'Bullying, depression and suicidal ideation in Finnish adolescents: school survey'. *British Medical Journal 319,* 350–448.

7. Rigby, K. and Slee, P.T. (1999) 'Suicidal ideation among adolescent school children, involvement in bully/victim problems and perceived low social support'. *Suicide and Life-threatening Behaviour 29,* 119–130.

8. Olweus, D. (1978) *Aggression in Schools. Bullies and Whipping Boys.* Washington, DC: Hemisphere Press (Wiley).

9. Huesmann, L.R., Eron, L.D., Lefkowitz, M.M. and Walder, L.O. (1984) 'The stability of aggression over time and generations'. *Developmental Psychology 20,* 1120–34.

10. Salmon, G., James, A. and Smith, D.M. (1998) 'Bullying in schools: Self reported anxiety, depression and self-esteem in secondary school children'. *British Medical Journal 317,* 924–925.

11. Salmon, G., James, A., Cassidy, E.L. and Javaloyes, M.A. (2000) 'Bullying a review: Presentations to an adolescent psychiatric service

and within a school for emotionally and behaviourally disturbed children'. *Clinical Child Psychology and Psychiatry 5*, 4, 1045–1359.

12. Tritt, C. and Duncan, R.D. (1997) 'The relationship between childhood bullying and young adult self-esteem and loneliness'. *Journal of Humanistic Education and Development 36*, 35–44.

13. Dietz, B. (1994) 'Effects on subsequent heterosexual shyness and depression on peer victimization at school'. Children's Peer Relations Conference. Adelaide: University of South Australia.

14. Olweus, D. (1992) 'Victimisation by peers: Antecedents and long term outcomes'. In K.H. Rubin and J.B. Asendorf (eds) *Social Withdrawal, Inhibition and Shyness in Children*. Hillsdale, NJ: Erlbaum.

15. Williams, K., Chambers, M., Logan, S. and Robinson, D. (1996) 'Association of common health symptoms with bullying in primary school children'. *British Medical Journal 313*, 17–19.

16. Rigby, K. (1998) 'The relationship between reported health and involvement in bully/victim problems among male and female secondary school students'. *Journal of Health Psychology 3*, 4, 465–476.

17. Rigby, K. (1999) 'Peer victimisation at school and the health of secondary school students'. *British Journal of Educational Psychology 69*, 95–104.

18. Forero, R., McLellan, L., Rissel, C. and Bauman, A. (1999) 'Bullying behaviour and psychosocial health among school students in New South Wales, Australia: Cross-sectional survey'. *British Medical Journal 319*, 344–348.

19. www.nas.org.uk/pubs/faqs/qbully.html

Childline in Partnerships with Schools
Studd Street
London N1 0QW
020 7239 1000
www.childline.org.uk

Further reading

Web addresses for further information and advice on bullying:

www.freecampus.co.uk/login/athome/parent/beyond/bullying.
index.htm

www.freecampus.co.uk/login/athome/parent/beyond/policies/
page07.htm (Webpages giving the equal opportunities policy of
Thurstable School including how to deal with bullies.)

www.nspcc.org.uk

www.bullyonline.org

www.bullying.co.uk

www.bully.org.uk

www.kidscape.org.uk

www.nas.org.uk/pubs/faqs/qbully.html (Advice on bullying from the
National Autistic Society.)

www.nobully.org.nz/guidelines.htm (Gives guidelines on how to
prevent bullying in school.)

Books

Elliot, M. (2002) *Bullying: A Practical Guide to Coping for Schools.* London:
    Pearson Education. (First published Longman 1991, then Financial
    Times Prentice Hall 1996.)
This book offers research into, and ways to cope with, the effects of bullying;
how to prevent bullying by learning to identify early signs and characteristics;
how to resolve difficult situations; offers advice to victims and helps children
become more self-confident, happy and open to learning.

Olweus, D. (1996) *Bullying at School.* Oxford: Blackwell Publishing. (First
    published 1993.)
This is a book written for adults containing much research material; suitable
for teachers and other professionals as well as parents.

Lindenfield, G. (1994) *Confident Children.* London: Thorsons.
This book has a section on bullying and the emphasis is on helping the child to
have high self-esteem and be able to protect him/herself.

Csóti, M. (2001) *Contentious Issues: Discussion Stories for Young People.* London: Jessica Kingsley Publishers.
This book consists of 40 discussion stories that challenge prejudice, stereotyping and judgemental behaviour, aimed at promoting awareness of others and challenging young people (aged 11 to 18) to consider events and the part they themselves play in life, helping them to become more responsible and independent thinking young adults. Bullying in various forms is addressed in a number of the discussion stories. It was designed for use in groups led by teachers, social workers or youth workers, but can easily be used by parents too.

Stones, R. (1993) *Don't Pick On Me! How to Handle Bullying.* London: Piccadilly Press.
This is an excellent book written in simple language for children to read. For those whose language skills are still in early stages, their parents can read it with them or tell them about it.

Lawson, S. (1994) *Helping Children Cope with Bullying.* London: Sheldon Press.
This is a book written for parents with much practical advice.

Rigby, K. (2002) *New Perspectives on Bullying.* London: Jessica Kingsley Publishers.
This is the most thorough of all the books (not only looking at bullying of children but also adults, including the elderly); covers a wider range of information and includes much research material. It is the most recommended text for professionals.

Csóti, M. (2001) *Social Awareness Skills for Children.* London: Jessica Kingsley Publishers.
This is a complete course in social skills training for children aged 7 to 16 including showing parents how to raise their child's self-esteem and teach assertiveness skills and confident body language.

Sharp, S. and Smith, P.K. (eds) (1994) *Tackling Bullying in your School: A Practical Handbook for Teachers.* London: Routledge.
This book provides a comprehensive guide to tackling bullying in schools including how to establish an anti-bullying policy, methods to tackle bullying during break times and methods for responding directly to bullying situations.

Goldman, J. (1995) *Sussed and Streetwise.* London: Piccadilly Press.
This book was written for teenagers to help keep them safe. It has a chapter on school that includes bullying and sexual harassment.

Chapter Four

Separation Anxiety

Separation anxiety is normal behaviour for toddlers aged six to eight months to three years and beyond. But for older children, particularly those who have been used to being left by their parents at nursery or friends' homes, to suddenly become anxious about separation again is not normal behaviour.

There may have been a crisis at home or a prolonged illness that the child has suffered that makes the child anxious again or she may have got used to being at home with her parents after a school holiday and miss the feeling of security it gave her.

Some children are anxious about being separated from their parents because of a particular problem they have, for example a disability or special educational needs such as an autistic spectrum disorder (see *Refusing school: children with autistic spectrum disorders* in Chapter One) and are afraid how others will react towards them or that they won't understand how to help them. It would help these children for the people around them to learn about the child's problems and what things help and what things make the problems (and hence anxiety) worse.

Signs of separation anxiety
A child is suffering from separation anxiety if she displays many of the signs described below:

- Becoming nervous about being left alone.

- Shadowing her parent.

- Getting nervous at the thought of her parent needing to leave.

- Not wanting to sleep alone.

- Having larger than usual fears of being burgled or of something lurking in a dark corner of her bedroom, or being convinced there's something horrible under her bed.

- Worrying that something will happen to her parent, or that her parent will leave her.

- Worrying that something will happen to her when away from her parent.

- Refusing to go to school.

- Having difficulty getting to sleep.

- Needing some light at night to see by, to check that her room is 'safe'.

- Having nightmares about becoming separated from her parent.

- Not wanting to be left at home alone (when at an age that this would be expected).

- Being afraid to go out without her parent.

- Experiencing physical symptoms of anxiety.

- Showing signs of distress when separation from her parent nears.

- Showing continuing signs of distress long after her parent has left.

With younger children, it is illegal for them to be left at home alone and it is natural that they should experience some anxiety about being left. However, if the child is desperately anxious when her parent just wants to pop something through the letterbox next door or to hang out washing, and the child is of school age, then there is a problem. Older children, who would normally be expected to be left at home alone but cannot, also have separation anxiety.

If the child is forced to do something she fears, she will show symptoms of panic and may even have a full-blown panic attack.

Very often, when a child is afraid of being in a certain environment, such as primary school, she may express a desire to regress and go back to the previous school, such as nursery. However, this is not to be recommended. The child must learn to cope in her current environment with her own peers (even if the environment needs to be adapted for a short while, such as the child attending the same school as her peers but being taught in a special unit).

The child needs to have explained that in life, things move on and do not go backwards and that she wouldn't have any of her friends at nursery if she were to return. Plus, she'd find what they do boring. Children need to be stimulated and have new things to do and learn, and it prepares them for their future. This is something distressed children do not want to think about, believing they will never leave home or want to. (I reassured my daughter, when she brought up the issue, that she could live at home forever if she wanted but also told her that when she is adult she probably won't want to.) This is not the time to impress upon a child that one day she will have to stand on her own two feet. She will often do that anyway if there is no pressure or expectation either way.

Risks of untreated separation anxiety

If a child has persistent fears about being separated from her parents and does not have professional help, she is at risk of having anxiety problems (such as agoraphobia) and panic disorder (see *Panic disorder and separation anxiety* in Chapter Two). Separation anxiety may persist into adulthood, making her life dependent and fraught and preventing her from leading a normal life.

Reducing the risks of the child developing separation anxiety

This section is useful for parents whose children already have school phobia, and for parents who have experienced it with one child and wish to prevent it occurring with another, although there are no guarantees; any number of things might happen to put a child off her stride.

However, being aware of some of the pitfalls might help reduce the risk and will certainly help support the child through her school career so that she finds school a positive and rewarding place to be.

This section can also be used to try to prevent a recurrence of the problem later in the child's school career, such as when she makes the transition from primary to secondary school. It is well documented that a child who has recovered from school phobia is at greater risk of the phobia recurring or of developing a worse school phobia in the future as she has already shown she is predisposed to this kind of anxiety.

In Chapter One, triggers of school phobia were mentioned; points 2 to 10 are dealt with in the pages following.

Starting school for the first time (primary)

Children aged four to five, starting school for the first time, are particularly susceptible to separation anxiety, so any fears they have about being separated from their main carers need to be allayed.

Anxiety can be reduced by regularly arranging for the child to play with other children when her parents are not there. They can send her to nursery and become involved with other parents so that their children are invited to the child's home and she to theirs. She needs to get used to being 'by herself' rather than being an extension of her parents. Getting used to other children's parents sharing the caring role prepares her for her teacher taking over when she starts school. This also prepares her for playing in different environments and learning to share toys with other children.

To reduce the child's anxiety about being in a strange environment, parents can visit the school with the child before she starts. Some nurseries arrange 'taster' sessions where the children spend a morning in their prospective school. Some also take their pupils to attend performances put on by the younger children of the school; or the child may be used to seeing, and being in, the school while picking up an older sibling with her parents or attending performances and sports days.

LEARNING ABOUT THE SCHOOL CULTURE AND EXPECTATIONS

The school 'culture' will be very different to what the child is used to. (The information below is from my own experience with primary schools.) For example, she needs to:

- Ask permission to go to the toilet.

- Be able to cope with visits to the toilet. Can the child wipe her bottom clean? Can the child cope with zips or buttons? (If not, parents will have to supply pull up trousers.) Can she cope with washing and drying her hands afterwards?

- Share the toys, pencils and rubbers, etc. with other children.

- Work in groups.

- Wait her turn.

- Tidy up after herself such as after cutting out shapes or painting.

- Be prepared to queue: at lunchtime; when the bell goes in the schoolyard; when the class is taken to the gym or to a music lesson; and at the end of the day before being given permission to leave.

- Cope with lunchtime etiquette:

    o having to sit in one place until lunch is eaten

    o being expected to eat even if she does not feel hungry

    o if having school dinners, needing to be able to carry a tray and to pick up a knife, fork, spoon and drink

    o having to ask for help from a stranger to cut up her food

    o eating food that might be strange to her

    o not spilling food and drink down her clothes

    o not dropping cutlery and food on the floor

    o having to stay when the others on the table get up to leave, because she hasn't finished her own food (however, not all dinner helpers stop the child, so some children might leave without having eaten much at all).

- Remember rules about not eating in class.

- Sit and listen when the teacher talks.

- Remember that if she wants to ask a question she must put up her hand and wait for the teacher to invite her to speak.

- Call the teacher 'Sir' or 'Miss' or by the teacher's name, such as Mrs Richards.

- Understand schoolyard etiquette: having to ask permission to join in other children's games rather than just expecting to; not running round corners as she might bump into someone; being careful where balls are thrown; and lining up quietly as soon as the bell is rung.

- Understand the meaning of the school bell. It indicates the start and end of things, depending on when it is rung. Sometimes it indicates the end of one thing and the start of the next – such as the end of the lesson and the start of break.

- Understand the instructions that are given.

- Understand what behaviour is unacceptable, such as fighting, hitting or spitting. Some behaviour is acceptable in the schoolyard, such as running and shouting, but is not acceptable inside the school building.

- Be able to cope with changing for games lessons and be prepared to ask for help if she can't do up her shoes on her own. (Parents could buy the child Velcro shoes or special plastic spiral laces that do not need to be tied.)

- Cope with a multitude of unexpected occurrences.

Parents should try to explain the differences that the child will come across so that they are not a complete shock to her. If possible, they could ask an older child who attends the same school what the day is like and what sort of things children have to remember.

Parents also need to help the child become as independent as she can so that she doesn't expect, or need, one-to-one help. This will give her the confidence to cope on her own when she is in school and learn to be responsible for herself.

Parents can help the child by carefully reading any literature that comes from the school:

- Is she expected to have done some preparatory work? If so, they should make sure it is done so that the child is not made to feel anxious about it in school. (For example, she might be expected to have learnt how to print the letters of the alphabet in the correct way or to recognise the sound of each letter.)

- Should all her clothes have name labels? This will help the teacher and the child: lost things will be easier to find, especially if the school has a uniform and all the clothes look the same. Can the child recognise her own clothes and shoes? If not, parents could play spotting games. For example, when friends come round and all the coats are together can the child spot her coat and her shoes, etc. quickly and accurately?

- Which day is dinner money day? (If parents send it in on the wrong day, the child will be told to take it home again, and she might be told off.)

If parents know an older child who goes to the same school, they could ask to look at the work done in his or her first year there. This will help them prepare the child for her tasks so that she finds school positive and rewarding rather than a place where she feels a failure.

If parents regularly role-play schools with the child, or if she plays schools with friends, it may help her be mentally prepared for the shift. If, for example, she sits at a table in the kitchen while a parent cooks, filling in a pre-school activity book (that is her 'work'), her parent can be the teacher directing her. If she wants help she must put up her hand and address the parent as 'Miss' or 'Sir'. It will also get her used to the idea of sitting in the same place for a fixed length of time doing 'work' – perhaps the only other time she sits in one place for any length of time is when she watches television.

THE SCHOOL'S TIMETABLE

The timing of the school day may present anxieties as it is very rigid and organised. The child might not be used to this, as life at home might be very relaxed, so she needs to have the timetable of the school day explained. For example, a typical primary school timetable might run like this:

1. At 8.50am the bell is rung in the schoolyard. All children line up with their class outside their particular entrance. The children are told when they can go in and on their way to their class have to take off and hang up their coats, hats, etc. and leave their bags and lunchboxes (if they have them) in the cloakroom. They may or may not be given particular pegs to use.

2. As soon as the class is seated and quiet (they may have to sit on the floor around the teacher), the teacher takes the register. They will be told how to answer when the teacher calls out their names. (For example, 'Yes, Miss' or 'Present'.)

3. The class may now go into assembly, quietly and in a line. They will be told where to sit in the hall. (Or assembly might be held later in the morning.)

4. After assembly, the children file quietly back to class and sit in their seats. The teacher gives them instructions on what to do next.

5. At 10.30am, it will be break time. All children are expected to go out into the schoolyard and play (the youngest children in the school often have their own schoolyard to play in to protect them from the rougher play of the older children). They are not allowed to stay in class (unless it is raining). They may eat fruit and have a drink (the class teacher will explain the rules). The children are expected to go to the toilet at break times so that they go as little as possible in class time; but children are always allowed to go to the toilet whenever they ask in the early years, as accidents are frequent.

6. At 10.50am, the bell will be rung and the children will have to line up again and wait to be told to go in. (This may be the time that they are given 'school milk'.) They should then sit at their tables and carry on with what they were doing before break or do whatever the teacher tells them to do next. Very often, when the children have finished their tasks, they can get out toys and play.

7. At about 11.50am, the children will be told to clear away and wash their hands for lunch. (They can go to the toilet if they wish.)

8. At 12pm, the bell sounds for lunch. The dinner helper might come to take the children in to lunch, children having school dinners at the front of the queue, children having sandwiches at the back, for example. Often, children having sandwiches have to sit at different tables to those having school dinners.

9. After lunch the children play in the schoolyard.

10. At 1pm, the bell is rung and the children will have to line up.

11. The afternoon may be spent painting or drawing or colouring pictures. It is usually less rigid than the morning. Or the children might learn ball skills, play outdoor games or dance.

12. At 2pm, the bell will sound for afternoon break. The children go outside and play. They can have a snack if they've brought one.

13. At 2.20pm, the bell will be rung for the children to line up again.

14. The children will be occupied with some activity until just before home time. They may have a story read to them.

15. At 3.20pm, the children will be told to clear everything away and get their bags, coats and lunchboxes (if they have them). Then they sit at their table to wait for the bell.

16. At 3.30pm the bell will be rung again and the children will join waiting parents or be filed out to get on a special school bus (in rural areas).

This is all a great deal for young children to take in. Much of their first term at school is spent socialising them. This involves getting them used to playing co-operatively with others and understanding the social structure of the school. Older children have more freedom and responsibility.

New children need to understand the role of class teachers, the headteacher, dinner helpers, caretaker and cleaners. Also, children need to learn what to do when, how to listen, how to tidy up after themselves and be responsible for their own books and other belongings, and where to keep their 'tray' to store their books.

Many children are slow at picking up new expectations and may be ridiculed, increasing their feeling of anxiety and making them very self-conscious. So any help with the above will increase the child's confidence.

BE ONLY POSITIVE

Parents should never say anything negative about the child's prospective school in front of her, even if they have heard bad things about it or they didn't have a good experience of schooling themselves. The school should only be shown in a positive light: they should tell the child it will be more interesting and fun or treat it as something of a non-event (this does not mean ignoring the impending change altogether), playing down the significance of the change and just informing the child of the expectation of her move. Parents could say, 'When you go to ... you can ...' without colouring it either way. Children tend to accept as the norm what their parents accept. (But they will need help in this; it will undo good work if parents' friends and relations give their spin on the prospective move to the child, such as saying, 'She's not going *there* is she?') The child doesn't need any worries before she starts school that she wouldn't have thought of herself. It is quite a difficult time for a child, stepping into the unknown, suddenly being among so many children and so many adults who she doesn't know or recognise. It will also be hard for her being the youngest, and probably one of the smallest, in the school after she has felt fairly grown-up and confident perhaps at nursery.

Another no-no is using the fact that the child is going to school as a threat or as a way to try to control inappropriate behaviour. Parents should not tell the child that she'd better watch out when she goes to school because the teachers won't be as understanding, or tell her that the teachers will sort her out because they are so strict. Comments like these are likely to make her fear going rather than seeing school as an exciting and adventurous step to take. (Sadly, in my daughter's school, the children were told before a move up to another class that they wouldn't get away with such behaviour with the next teacher and that they'd better look out. If it really is true, the more challenging children will find out soon enough: the timid ones don't need to know.)

Parents should try to prevent older children, such as children of friends of theirs, older siblings or slightly older friends of the child, telling her stories about school that could make her anxious.

Parents should make a big fuss of the child and tell her how proud they are of her for being ready to start school. They could buy her a special present to mark the occasion, for after her first day at school, letting her know this will happen well in advance so that she looks forward to the present before she starts school and so that the anticipation can help distract her from any possible anxieties.

Also before school starts, the child will need basic equipment and possibly a school uniform. Parents can take her shopping so that she can choose a school bag, lunchbox, pencil case, etc. and tell her that these are not for now: they are for when she starts school. This will again help her associate going to school with nice things.

Parents can tell the child what new things she can look forward to at school, such as a playhouse and many more toys and friends to play with when she's finished her work. If she likes art, she can look forward to spending more time doing it in more interesting ways. Her class may also have a computer for her to try. They also often watch educational children's programmes on the television.

COMMUNICATION SKILLS NEEDED FOR STARTING SCHOOL

Children can feel anxious about being separated from a parent because they do not have the necessary communication skills to function away from him or her. This may be because of a particular medical condition such as an autistic spectrum disorder. (See *Refusing school: children with autistic spectrum disorders* in Chapter One.) For example, if the child's speech is indistinct, parents are well practised at deciphering the words and can quickly understand her needs. But a teacher might not be able to. This can cause the child great anxiety, feeling that it is only her parents who can meet her needs.

When the child goes to school she needs to be able to communicate effectively with other children and the adults who care for her, particularly her class teacher:

1. Can the child explain her needs? (Can she, for example, ask to go to the toilet or tell someone she doesn't feel well?)

2. Can her speech be understood? (If her speech is unclear, people will have trouble understanding her and this can cause great difficulties and misunderstandings, particularly if the child is unable to put them right.)

3. Is the child too shy to speak to people in authority such as her class teacher?

4. Can the child listen effectively so that she can understand instructions and act on them?

All the above points are vital to the child feeling at ease within the school environment. If she feels that the only people she can communicate with are her parents she will feel miserable when in school because she will feel misunderstood and isolated from those around her.

HELPING THE CHILD TO BE ABLE TO EXPLAIN HER NEEDS

It is vital that the child can explain her needs to the class teacher and dinner helper and to ask for help when needed. To practise verbal communication with the child at home, parents must not anticipate her needs by doing things for her or by asking, 'Would you like to go outside to play now?' This is an example of a 'closed' question because it requires only a 'yes' or 'no' answer or a nod or shake of the head, or the child might just go and play without saying a word. Parents should encourage the child to express herself by asking, 'What would you like to do now?' This is an example of an 'open' question, requiring the child to make up her own mind and giving her more opportunity for verbal communication. Examples of other open questions are:

- 'What would you like to do today?'
- 'What would you like for tea?'
- 'What do you want to wear today?'
- 'What shall we do first?'

To increase verbal communication after the child has done something such as painting a picture, parents could ask her to tell them about what she's done, why she chose certain colours and whether she's pleased with her efforts ('What do you think of it?').

Parents should regularly ask the child's opinion, generally, by asking questions such as: What did she like about the television programme she's just watched? What didn't she like?

Another way to improve the child's communication skills is for parents to frequently ask her to report back on what she's done or where she's been, such as: how was the meal, her trip to the shops, the stay at her friend's home? This can be a hard skill for children as they have to use the past tense. They also need to relate the event in a logical sequence. If the child cannot do this, parents could prompt her by saying, 'What did you do first of all?'

As well as improving her skills, this helps protect her so that if anything bad happens when she is away from her parents, she can tell them about it. It is a good idea for parents always to ask how the child's school day went when she gets home and spend some time together with no distractions. This may then act as an early warning when trouble is brewing. However, many children don't divulge much about their day. When asked about what they did they might shrug and say, 'Nothing much'.

Sometimes it is the particular words the child uses that cause incomprehension such as pet family euphemisms that other adults and children may not understand. Baby talk (such as using 'narna' for 'banana') should also be discouraged.

IMPROVING THE CHILD'S SPEECH

If there are particular sounds or words that the child finds hard to say, parents could practise saying them with her. They could try rewarding her for her efforts by having a Lego block awarded to a pot every time she says the sound correctly, as well as giving praise and cuddles and applause. They will know whether the reward has hit home by the way the child reacts. If she shows pleasure at how she is treated and indicates through body language that she is proud of herself, the reward is working.

When there are 20, 50 or 100 Lego blocks in the pot, parents could reward her with something she has looked forward to for some time or do something special with her. (They should discuss the reward with the child so that she has input and feels in control about what happens, which will help raise her self-esteem and motivate her.)

If the child has a definite speech problem that parents don't feel able to correct, they should ask her doctor to refer her to a speech therapist and ask the therapist how best to help her at home.

IMPROVING THE CHILD'S ABILITY TO TALK TO PEOPLE IN AUTHORITY

Young children's shyness can be all consuming and they can be so overcome that they are unable to initiate speech with an unfamiliar adult. If the child is like this, the best way to get around it is to try and immerse her in speech with many different adults. Some suggestions for parents are:

- Remind the child to say 'Thank you' and 'Goodbye', etc. at the appropriate times so that she can eventually say these things without being prompted. Reward her with a Lego block (see above) every time she remembers to do this herself.

- Ask the child to give simple messages to her friends' parents.

- Ask friends to speak to the child as much as possible so that she feels comfortable speaking to them and is encouraged to initiate conversation herself. (She can, for example, tell them about her pet or where she's been or what item of clothing she's recently been bought.) Parents need to ensure they don't answer for her, even if there's a pause while the child thinks. If she's too shy, needing further prompting, they could say to her, 'Repeat what you told me about...'

- Let the child see that sharing news with others is a natural event. If she hears her parents updating friends on what they've done and they invite her to chip in, she's more likely to feel at ease doing it on her own in the future.

- Let the child pay for simple items in shops (her parent could stand next to her to help her if she needs it and to make her feel secure while doing it).

- Let the child ask a shop assistant if, for example, the shop stocks yo-yos (her parent could stand next to her).

The child could be rewarded with Lego blocks every time she does a 'brave' thing such as speaking to another adult (but she should be reminded that she should only speak to adults she does not know when accompanied by a parent, for safety reasons). It is vital the child gets rewarded in a positive way to motivate her to continue making the effort.

HELPING THE CHILD LISTEN EFFECTIVELY SO THAT SHE CAN UNDERSTAND INSTRUCTIONS AND ACT ON THEM

Parents can practise giving simple instructions to the child such as, 'Can you fetch me the purple box that's on the floor by my bed?' If the child can cope with these, parents could try harder ones such as, 'Will you bring down the yellow jumper that's on the left hand shelf in Daddy's wardrobe?'

A way to check effective listening is by reading a story to the child and then asking her about it. Parents can also extend her skills by asking things that were not in the story such as, 'Why do you think he did that?' or 'Can you think of a better way to have got it back?'

PHYSICAL SKILLS NEEDED FOR STARTING SCHOOL

Some children have motor skills problems because of a medical condition such as dyspraxia and autistic spectrum disorders (see *Refusing school: children with autistic spectrum disorders* in Chapter One) that make it even harder for them to acquire the skills mentioned below. They will

need more time and more practice than other children to learn both fine
motor skills (such as tying shoelaces and handwriting) and gross motor
skills (such as running, skipping, jumping, catching and kicking). Can
the child:

- Dress and undress herself?

- Cope with her toilet needs?

- Hold a pencil correctly?

- Copy shapes and write letters of the alphabet?

- Draw pictures?

- Colour in pictures that she's drawn or that are in colouring
  books? Does she know that she should try to keep inside the
  lines? Parents should make sure she has the appropriate
  equipment for the job. (For example, if the picture needs fine,
  detailed colouring, the child will need a sharp colouring
  pencil: thick stubby crayons are more suited to colouring big
  expanses, and felt pens can smudge and make a mess.)

- Join dot-to-dot pictures? If they are numbered, this will help
  her counting skills.

- Trace over pictures? Greaseproof paper can be used in the
  absence of tracing paper. (Some activity books involve
  tracing and are sold with leaves of tracing paper in the
  appropriate places in the book.)

- Run, hop, skip and jump? She will be expected to be able to
  do this in gym lessons.

- Skip with a rope? She might be too young yet as this is
  difficult to do, but it is part of schoolyard culture so she
  could start to learn. Boys need to skip too for sports day,
  even if they feel it is a girl's game for the schoolyard. If they
  are reluctant, it could be pointed out that men use skipping
  ropes in fitness training.

- Play with a yo-yo? Although, like skipping, this is quite a
  hard skill to master and may need to wait a year or two, it

does no harm to introduce it and have it available for the
child to pick up if she wants to.

- Kick and catch balls? She will be expected to do this in 'ball
  skills' at school and will need some ball control skills for
  sports day.

- Balance and walk on a low wall? She will be expected to do
  this on a bench in gym lessons.

- Step only on the cracks in pavements? This is akin to
  stepping-stones.

The child may well not have all these skills when she starts school, but
just having some and working on the rest will help her feel confident.
There will be plenty of other children, at least for the first year or two,
that need help with, for example, shoes and buttons.

Starting school for the first time (secondary)

For the first time, the child may need to travel on public transport to
school or walk a long way or even cycle to school. She should practise
the route several times (or even try out several routes to find out which
she prefers) so that she is confident about the journey and how long it
will take. If the child is to use public transport, parents could get a copy
of the relevant timetable so that she knows when the next train or bus
will be if she misses her usual one or if it is cancelled (or teach the child
to read the timetable displayed at the bus stop, for example).

It is also important for the child to have the right uniform and sports
kit and have accessories (such as rain jacket and school bag) that are
similar to those the others at the school have. It will help her fit in and be
included.

Although children may be well used to a school environment, it is
nevertheless a big change going from primary to secondary school and
it would be good for parents to tell them about some of the differences
they can expect so that the change is not so daunting or such a shock to
them.

Ideally the child's parents should talk to other parents who have
children in the same secondary school and have her talk to a pupil of

that school too. Some things that are different in secondary school are (from personal experience):

- The school will be much bigger: some schools have as many as 2000 pupils on roll.

- There is likely to be more than one building. Some schools have several buildings or a couple of main buildings plus mobile classrooms.

- The buildings may have staircases (only new modern schools are built on one level to be accessible by the disabled).

- The child will have to learn the routes from each class to the next and find out where the toilets, dining hall and assembly hall are. (Many schools issue new pupils with a plan of the school to help them.) It helps the child if she has visited the school before.

- Some schools have split sites where the pupils may have a five to ten minute walk between. However, usually the older children and the staff 'commute' while the younger children stay on the same site. This can be beneficial to younger children as they are effectively in a smaller school with fewer staff, with children only up to three years older. They may be based there for three years before they move on to the upper school. The downsides are that they don't have the benefit of having sensible older children and prefects as role models and they effectively have to get used to a new school when they make the transition to the upper school.

- There can be well over 100 teachers in the school so the child will not recognise most of the staff to begin with and certainly won't know all their names. Likewise, not all the staff will know the child.

- There will probably be a majority of male staff (in UK primary schools the majority of teachers are women). The child may never have had a man teach her before.

- The child will be given a form room that she shares with others in the same form, where registration takes place with her form teacher. She will have the same form teacher for the whole year. (Some schools like continuity, so the form teacher may be with the child for several years.) Generally forms stay the same so the child won't have to worry about being with different children at the start of each school year.

- Registration takes place twice a day. Some schools have form room registration only once, in the afternoon, the morning registration being carried out during the first lesson by the subject teacher.

- Assembly may be in the morning or the afternoon. If form room registration takes place in the afternoons only, assembly will follow that.

- There might not be assembly every day as some schools have only one assembly hall, which might not be big enough to accommodate the whole school. Thus, certain years may be grouped to have assembly, say, twice a week.

- If the child has problems, she can talk to her form teacher about them or the Head of Year (heads of year are involved in disciplinary measures and pastoral care).

- Form teachers don't take dinner money. Usually children pay at the canteen where they get their lunch. Some schools have children buy dinner vouchers from a school secretary or use 'smart' cards that can be topped up every few weeks with a cheque from home.

- The child will have to be responsible for what she chooses to eat at the canteen if it is one where she pays for the items she chooses with cash or a 'smart' card, rather than using a voucher system that buys a complete lunch.

- There won't be dinner helpers as there are in primary schools. Secondary school children are expected to be able to cut their own food and not need encouragement to eat up.

- Children are expected to move from class to class instead of the teacher coming to them. For example, maths may be taught in the maths block and science in the science block and so on. Some teachers may move classrooms or laboratories too to share certain facilities with other members of the department. For example, there may be only two physics laboratories but three classes of physics taught at the same time. So use of the laboratories would have to be rotated to enable each class to have the opportunity to carry out experiments. So if, for example, the child has physics on Tuesdays and Fridays, she may be in the laboratory on Tuesday but in a classroom on Friday. So she will need to put rooms as well as subjects on her timetable so that she knows where to go for each lesson.

- Lessons aren't all taught using form groupings. Maths and English may be banded, for example, so that the children are grouped with others of similar ability. Later in the child's school career, when she is starting her GCSE courses, her timetable will be individual to her and she may be in a different class to her best friend all the time, apart from games/PE.

- The child will no longer be at the top of the school but at the bottom due to her age.

- The child may only know a small number of children in the school as secondary schools can have many primary feeder schools.

- The older children will be much bigger and may seem intimidating.

- If the school has a sixth form, there may be prefects. Prefects help teachers with gate and break duties and they may help organise the queues at lunchtimes.

- The child will probably be given a homework timetable (on which days she'll be given homework for which subjects) and a diary where she has to write down her homework. Parents are expected to sign this at the end of the week. (Probably only 20 to 30 minutes' homework is given for each double lesson the child has in her first year, and she should be given more than one night to complete it.)

- The child will not have a tray where she keeps her work. She will have to carry all her books, etc. around with her. Some schools provide lockers.

- The child must check her timetable and make sure she has the right books for the right day and adequate writing equipment. Secondary school teachers do not stock spare pens and pencils, etc. and the child will get into trouble if she does not have writing equipment with her.

- The child will have more subjects to learn about, many of which she may not have heard about before. This can be exciting as it opens up new areas of interest to the child and she has a chance to make a fresh start.

- The child will not be allowed to go to the toilet during lessons (unless she has a medical problem). She must make sure she goes at break time.

- The child will be expected to stay seated while putting up her hand to ask a question rather than walking up to the teacher. (Shouting out is not allowed: the child must wait to be invited to speak.)

- The child will be expected to know where to start each day's work in her book. The teacher will tell her soon after she joins the class if she is to underline the previous lesson's work or to start a new page for each new topic. She is not then expected to ask at the start of each lesson where she should write her first word.

- The child will be expected to listen, understand and remember safety rules of the environment she is in, such as when in science lessons. Here, for example, she is expected to wear safety goggles and tie back long hair whenever Bunsen burners are used and know how to safely carry a lighted splint. She will also need to remember never to run in a laboratory and always to tuck her bag under the bench or table so that it doesn't trip someone up.

- There may be numerous after-school clubs to join, which could be fun.

- The school may have a homework club where the child can go to do her homework in an atmosphere of quiet, and there may be someone on hand to help her.

- There will be regular testing in school. Sometimes the tests are small ones, but probably at the end of each year the child will be set 'exams' when she has to sit and work through specially prepared papers under strict supervision.

- The child may see undesirable behaviour such as children smoking, making rude signs, fighting, shouting at the teacher, refusing to co-operate and vandalising things by breaking them or defacing them with graffiti.

It may help to find out if the school has a strong anti-bullying policy so that parents know if the school takes it seriously and is prepared to confront bullying and bullies rather than dismiss it, not wanting to get involved.

Parents might like to point out to the child that some things will be the same as in her previous school, such as:

- The school day will be organised by the sounding of bells. (Teachers won't ring a hand bell, however, and the children don't line up outside – they just go to the next lesson.)

- Children are still expected to go outside or sit in cloakrooms (if it is raining) at break times.

- There will always be a member of staff on duty at break times and lunchtimes should there be a problem.

- Reports will be sent home (but up to three times a year).

- There will be a parents' evening to find out how the child is doing. Parents will need to see each subject teacher involved with the child but may not need to see the form teacher unless there's a specific problem he or she should know about.

Moving to a new area, having to join a new school and make new friends or just changing schools

Whenever a child changes school, there is bound to be some anxiety as every school has a different feel to it and the atmosphere will be different. The rules may have to be relearnt (some schools ban chewing gum or all sweets, for example) and so the child needs to be prepared for things to feel strange for a while.

If possible, parents should invite new friends round as soon as the child shows a preference for one or two or can tell her parents with whom she regularly sits. If parents go to school to pick up the child, it would be useful to chat to the parents of other children in the child's class to help identify which children like their child, and make it easier to invite other children round.

Even if the child has changed from an infant to a junior school (or in some areas from a first to a middle school), some rules and expectations may change. They can change again for the transition to secondary school.

Being off school for a long time through illness or because of a holiday

Children who have learnt about and have happily experienced the school environment may have anxiety following a long break from school, whether because of a summer holiday or absence due to illness.

A long holiday break can make children dread the return to school where they feel less at home and secure under the scrutiny of peers and teachers. There is not much that can be done here other than for parents to support the child for the first few days back at school and, if possible, invite school friends for her to play with before she goes back to school so that the bonding process is reinforced and can continue in school hours. (This is easier if the family doesn't go away for the entire holiday, and nor do the child's friends.)

If the child has been ill, she may have become used to a great deal of attention, particularly if it has been a protracted illness where a great deal of care was needed. The extra attention she has needed should be gradually withdrawn as soon as she no longer needs it. She should also be encouraged to return to normal activities within the home as soon as she is able, to escape the idea that she is sick and helpless. She needs to regain her independence and with it her confidence.

Bereavement (of a person or pet)

Finding out that life does not go on without change can be a very daunting experience to any child, but particularly to a sensitive and fragile child. And to find out through practical experience rather than theoretically, as in a story, can be very disturbing. The child has to come to terms with the fact that the same thing could happen to someone very close to her (if it hasn't already) and she may fear family members, particularly her main carer, dying and being left alone with no one to look after or comfort her.

Parents should try to explain to her why her pet or grandparent, for example, has died. Knowing about old age and the serious illnesses that may come with it may help her feel less anxious, as she understands that her parents are not likely suddenly to have, for example, a massive stroke that kills them.

Bereavement is harder to handle if it concerns the death of another child. However, a simple explanation of why it has happened may help, as the child can then ponder over whether it is likely to happen to her or to someone close to her. If she is worried that death is commonplace among the young, parents can remind her of all the children in her school who she knows and ask how many of them she has heard of dying. Talking to her about these things helps her get death into perspective.

If parents think it appropriate, they could watch a programme like *Animal Hospital* with the child so that she can see for herself what miracles vets can perform and understand why they are sometimes unsuccessful. (It is important an adult watches with the child to gauge her reaction and dispel any wrong ideas she may have. It also provides insight into what her fears are if she can question adults about what she has seen.) Learning about life through a programme on pets is likely to be less daunting than watching medical programmes, which is not advised. For example, *Children's Hospital* can be extremely distressing and may introduce unfounded fears about medical problems and the hospital environment.

Feeling threatened by the arrival of a new baby

It is an immense shock for a child who is used to much one-to-one attention from her parents when a baby comes along, particularly if there is a big age gap. If possible, parents should try to put time aside to spend with the child when she gets home from school or when the parents get home from work (parents might be able to have the baby amused in his or her playpen or asleep in another room), so that she has their undivided attention. Perhaps the baby can be fed separately so that family mealtimes remain as they were (as far as is possible with a demanding baby). At bedtime, parents should try to be separately involved with the child, if there are two, so that the child has a continuing one-to-one relationship with each, is reassured of her status in the family home and does not feel pushed aside because of the new baby. She will then feel less resentful of her new sibling and may enjoy getting involved by helping at bath time or during the baby's meals.

Having a traumatic experience such as being abused, being raped, having witnessed a tragic event

Parents should be aware that any distressing event may have a bad effect on the child, including a home fire or burglary or being in, or witnessing, a road accident. If she looks preoccupied and does not seem as happy as usual, parents should either talk to her about what has happened or try to find out what is troubling her if they don't already know. If parents cannot get to the bottom of what is troubling the child, is there a chance that someone is abusing her? Whoever might be abusing her will need help, as will the child. The abuser also poses a risk to other children while he or she is still at large in the community.

Witnessing something very disturbing such as a fatal accident can trigger post-traumatic stress disorder (PTSD) (see Chapter Two) in susceptible children. Any child who has seen things a child does not normally see is at risk in the same way. If lesser anxiety-causing events are not handled carefully they may also lead to PTSD in a susceptible child, whereas in others they may not. For example, had I initially handled the fire alarm problem (see *Introduction*) in a calm and matter-of-fact way, my daughter may not have been so disturbed about the subsequent alarms, but there are no guarantees. Parents can help children with PTSD in the following ways:

- They should not be afraid of expressing personal fears. This encourages the child to talk of her own fears and not bottle them up; she will see how her parents cope with their own fears, encouraging her to do the same.

- They should accept the child's fears and talk about them freely. Discussion helps her put her fears into perspective and helps her find her own way through. Parents don't have to have all the answers; it will comfort her to know that someone cares enough to listen to her and take her seriously. And she won't feel so isolated or alone.

- They should help the child put her fears into perspective. Young children cannot think logically and some older ones may be too caught up in the traumatic event to do so. Parents can help correct distorted beliefs (such as a child believing that the world is a very dangerous place) by applying her experience to everyday common occurrences. They can test the child's logic underlying her belief so that she can see that she has lost perspective.

- They should relate traumatic events to probability at a level the child can understand. For example, when my daughter was worried about breaking another bone after breaking her wrist, I told her that if bones were so easily broken, half the population would be wearing a cast, and how many people did she know that wore one? When she was anxious about going on a ferry, thinking it might sink and having heard about the film *Titanic*, I told her that thousands of safe crossings are completed each year so the likelihood (and in the summer when the sea is calmer than the winter) was tiny.

- They should limit the child's exposure to other traumatic events by not allowing her to watch the news or violent programmes or films (including 'disaster movies'). This may be hard following 11 September and other much-talked-of terrorist attacks, especially if the child has been closely involved in some way.

- They should be physically and verbally affectionate towards the child. This is a time when she very much needs to feel loved, comforted and secure.

If necessary, parents should seek counselling or get advice from a professional. Bad experiences can have far-reaching effects and it is vital that the child is handled sensitively and appropriate help is found. There may be reasons why parents would like to forget about the traumatic incident as quickly as possible, but this is not helpful to the child. Even if parents think she may have forgotten about, for example, being abused, there is sufficient evidence to suggest this is probably not so. Brushing it under the carpet doesn't get rid of it – it'll come out sooner or later.

Problems at home such as a member of the family being very ill

Problems at home can give the child stress. Parents will need to explain to her what is happening in such a way that they relieve her fears and make her feel more secure. Fear of the unknown can cause much distress and, without talking to the child, parents will not know how she has interpreted the various scenes and the snippets of conversations she has overheard.

Parents should be aware of the child and the distress she might be experiencing, and try to relieve it. If, for example, one of her parents has an illness that obviously interferes with everyday life and is noticeable within the home, the nature of the illness should be explained in simple words to relieve the child's worry. Telling her everything is fine when it isn't will not convince the child and will only make her keep her anxieties to herself – she will probably believe that either her parents don't want to talk to her about the situation and are deliberately shutting her out, or that it is too serious to be talked about and that something bad might happen.

Problems at home such as marital rows, separation and divorce

Marital rows can disturb children and make them feel insecure, as they may see and hear things that they don't understand or that make them feel unsafe. They may be asked to take sides but feel the need to show allegiance to both parents. They may be asked to comfort a parent, which can be distressing because their experience of family life may have been that they were always the comforted ones up until then. They may feel as if they are to blame when an upset parent pushes them away or cannot comfort them when they need help, understanding and support themselves.

If parents are going through separation or divorce, their child may feel insecure, fearing abandonment, and she may feel guilty in some way, thinking it is her fault (as many children do) even though it probably has nothing to do with her. Parents should explain to their child what is going to happen, that it isn't in any way her fault, and that they both still love her very much. They should try to avoid rowing in her presence and allow the child to be loyal to both of them.

Violence in the home or any kind of abuse of the child or another parent or carer

Being abused can traumatise a child. If the child sees a parent being abused, she may be too frightened to leave that parent, believing something bad might happen while she is not there. The violence or abuse needs to be addressed before the child can be expected to feel happier and more secure.

Conclusion

Life is full of pitfalls and it is the job of a parent to try to anticipate the effect these may have on the child and to reassure and comfort the child when she is distressed. It is also the job of a parent to equip the child with the necessary confidence and skills to eventually cope on her own so that she can lead a full and satisfying life of her choosing. This is no easy task, but is helped by allowing the child freedom to develop in a secure and calm environment (where she does not have to fear harsh or inconsistent discipline), at her own pace and by not being over-protected. If the child shows a desire to do new things on her own then, unless it is still dangerous for any child of her age, she should be allowed to go ahead.

Healing a child of separation anxiety is allowing her to be set free; the parent needs to learn to let go at the appropriate time for the child, while encouraging her in the process. And, if the parent's presence makes no difference to the outcome of the child's anxiety (such as when

I stayed in school to help my daughter relax but found my presence made no difference), that presence is redundant (regardless of whether the child asks for it). Over-fussing does not help, but makes matters worse. The child may as well be on her own and develop the confidence to know that, whatever happens, she can manage the situation herself.

Further reading

Web addresses on separation anxiety:

www.aacap.org/publications/factsfam/anxious.htm (From the American Academy of Child and Adolescent Psychiatry.)

npin.org/pnews/2000/pnew500/feat500.html (National Parent Information Network in the US.)

www.mentalhealth.com/fr00.html (Mental health website with a detailed index.)

Woolfson, R. (1995) *Starting School*. London: Thorsons.
This is a very practical book for parents about getting their (under five) child ready for first school, including chapters for children with special needs and on common problems in the infant class.

Chapter Five

Social Phobia

The second type of school phobia is social phobia. For a child to be diagnosed with social phobia, she must show that she does have social relationships appropriate to her age with familiar people and her anxiety must appear in peer settings, not just in interactions with adults. Although adults with social phobia know that their fear is unreasonable, children may not; they may not even understand what causes their fear (not being able to identify irrational thoughts), only knowing they must avoid certain social situations.[1]

In school, children suffering from social phobia may be frightened of being criticised and evaluated by, or humiliated in front of, their peers. Assemblies and school performances can cause great anxiety: the children may have to read out loud or take part in a drama scene. Simply attending assemblies may create anxiety because there is no escape and the children are scrutinised by teachers and the headteacher. Sometimes children with social phobia may fear fainting in assembly if the pupils have to stand instead of sit. Frequently, children with social phobia fear having to eat in public.

The classroom environment may also cause stress. The children may be afraid of being asked a question in front of the rest of the class (and fear being ridiculed should they give the wrong answer) or having to read out loud (fearing they will stammer and stumble over words or not pronounce them correctly and be laughed at).

Physical activities can also cause stress, where children feel they are being evaluated for their physical skills. They may fear dropping the ball they're supposed to catch, coming last in a race or being one of the last to be picked for a team.

Children with social phobia fear unpopularity with their peers and are highly sensitive to any form of rejection whether real or perceived. This fear of rejection is made worse if the child has parents with very high expectations or who are highly critical of her. The slightest negative feeling a child gets from someone else can stay with her all day and beyond.

Children suffering from social phobia isolate themselves from others, being too anxious about rejection to form positive relationships and to initiate conversation with others. This affects the way they feel about school and their performance in school: a stressed child cannot learn well.

Social phobic children are also anxious about social interactions with authority figures (such as teachers, doctors and nurses) and other adults (being of an age where they would have already developed relationships with their peers and familiar adults).

Social phobia and shyness

Social phobia is not shyness; some adults with social phobia are very outgoing and only experience anxiety in specific social situations such as public speaking or having to use a public toilet. However, the majority of children who suffer from social phobia are also shy and lacking in social skills (adults can hide discomfort more easily than children, can act confident even when they aren't, and have had more practice with social skills). The social phobic child will go to enormous lengths to avoid a threatening situation, whereas the shy child might just feel awkward and uncomfortable for a while but wouldn't refuse to go.[1]

The reason only socially phobic children actively avoid social situations is because of the extreme levels of anxiety they experience. A child with social phobia might completely freeze and be unable to say or do anything. She might suffer a panic attack or symptoms of intense anxiety that are related to panic such as crying, throwing a tantrum or shrinking away from the event or person.[1] A shy child does not experience such high levels of anxiety.

Another difference between shyness and social phobia is that shyness develops early in life and many children grow out of it. The predominant age of onset for social phobia is between 11 and 15 years.[2]

Theories behind social phobia and shyness

Shyness can be considered to be of two types: fearful shyness and self-conscious shyness.[3] Fearful shyness is an extension of behavioural inhibition (first mentioned in *Why do panic attacks start?* in Chapter Two) where children show fear, caution and withdrawal in novel situations to keep them safe from strangers. Children who have persistent behavioural inhibition have been found to experience, when in a novel situation, physiological changes in their body that correspond to those changes produced when afraid. In other words, they have a very sensitive nervous system (thought to be genetic and a possible explanation of why anxiety disorders run in families).

Self-conscious shyness is thought to develop much later than fearful shyness as it needs a sense of self to exist that very young children don't have. Self-conscious awareness involves the child being able to see herself from an observer's point of view (public awareness) and having negative thoughts about herself that tie in with how she thinks others see her. When public awareness is acute, the child feels conspicuous and embarrassed.

Other models of shyness have been used in research, but whichever model a researcher proposes, it is thought that the combined effects of the two types of shyness are cumulative in their effect, predisposing a child to social phobia if both are present.

Selectively mute (see entry later in the chapter) children are believed to be a subset of inhibited children who have not learnt to quiet their nerves in social interaction.[4]

Social phobia: children with autistic spectrum disorders

Children with autistic spectrum disorders can have much experience of being rejected and ridiculed (because of their problems in socialising and sometimes in their lack of motor skills, more obvious in games and PE), which can make them dread social interactions, leading to social phobia.

Some children with autistic spectrum disorders would like to have a friend and would appreciate help in achieving that. Others like to spend time on their own and should not be forced to socialise if they are happy and less stressed when alone.

Being with other children and taking part in social interactions will help children with autistic spectrum disorders, but this should only be done with the child's co-operation in a way that is acceptable to the child and in an environment that is least likely to cause stress. Each child needs to be considered as an individual; the key point here is that these children suffer extreme anxiety and so caution is required at every stage not to intensify this.

Onset of social phobia

Very often, there is a gradual onset of unease and a gradual build-up of tension in social situations and the child may not suffer full-blown social phobia (with panic attacks) until later on in her teens. Full-blown social phobia for adolescent sufferers aged 14 to 16 (see later in this chapter) can include problems and fears additional to those of younger sufferers.

Children over age eight can suffer from social phobia even though other anxieties (such as agoraphobia and separation anxiety) still exist. Below are considered the trigger points of school phobia for children over age eight that were mentioned in Chapter One, points 11 to 13, relating to social anxiety.

Not having good friends (or any friends at all)

Friends are vital to everyone for support, affection, companionship, people to do things with and sharing experiences. Friends give children a sense of belonging, of inclusion within a group where they have a place, are respected and their opinions and company sought.

No child likes to be thought friendless as it implies a lack of status, having no one to care about her. It is also emotionally painful when a child sees other children together and having fun while she is left out.

For a child to feel good about herself, have high self-esteem and be confident, she needs to have her presence valued. It is safer for children to have a small group of friends who can socialise with one another than a single 'best' friend who may suddenly become someone else's best friend, be off sick for a long time or leave the area: then the child is left abandoned, unable to function without this other half. It is up to parents to encourage the child to have as wide a circle of friends as possible, and they can help by inviting friends round or including friends in family outings such as to the local swimming pool or cinema.

Joining clubs in school time and after school can help children have interests in common with other children. The more opportunity for social interaction, the better the child will become and the more comfortable she will feel, increasing her confidence. Ideas to help a child maintain her friendships could include the following:

- When a friend is ill, the child could ring up to find out how he or she is. Or she could make a 'Get Well' card to take round or post, or send an electronic card by email.

- If the child is bored or lonely on the weekend, she could ring up or call on a friend to invite him or her round.

- Parents can share lifts to clubs with other parents so that the child always arrives with another child and is used to being taken around by other adults.

- The child could send friends postcards when she is on holiday. For closer friends, she could buy them a small gift such as a bookmark or a souvenir pen.

- When a friend has a music or drama exam, the child could ring her up or make her a card, to wish her luck.

- When a friend has received good news the child should congratulate her.

- Basic friendship rules could be explained to the child to help her make fewer mistakes such as (taken from page 75 of my book, *Social Awareness Skills for Children*):

    o Keep your friends' secrets (unless doing so puts them in danger).

    o Never tell lies about your friend.

    o Don't try to deliberately get your friend into trouble (for example, because you are jealous of something).

- o Don't be rude or horrible to a friend without apologising afterwards and explaining why you said the things you did.

- o Don't let your friend do all the running. If he's always the one that calls for you, you should sometimes show him that you want his company too by calling on him.

- o Keep the relationship balanced by offering to help your friend when he's in trouble – not expecting him to be the one that helps you without reciprocating.

- o Don't be jealous of the time your friend spends with others. It's healthier to have more than one friend, and being over-possessive loses you friends and makes you unhappy. Develop other friendships or interests yourself.

Things the child can do to make new friends (taken from page 76 of my book, *Social Awareness Skills for Children*):

- Go up and say 'hello'.

- Ask the person's name.

- Tell her your name.

- Ask her something to do with the place you're in, such as: 'Is this your first time at the club?', 'Have you been camping before?', 'Where was your old school?' or 'Why did you change school?'

- Give information at the same level about yourself. For example, if she tells you how old she is, tell her your age.

- Offer to do something for the person. For example, you could offer to show her round the school, sit by her at lunch, share a toy or invite her to join in your game.

- Ask her to help you in some way. ('Can you help me do…?') Then you can start chatting – about what you need help with, and later other things too.

Parents can help their child make new friendships by:

- Inviting children round to the home.

- Suggesting conversation openers the child could use, such as 'Where do you live? How long have you lived there?' or 'Can you tell me what I should do about...?' or 'What are the school dinners like?' or 'Do you go to Scouts? What sort of things do you do?'

(Also see *Dealing with shyness and making new friends,* later in the chapter.)

Being unpopular, being chosen last for teams and feeling a physical failure (in games and gymnastics)

Where possible, parents could improve the child's skills by getting her involved in clubs after school. With tuition and practice, she should improve and feel less of a failure when with her classmates. Physical fitness and confidence in performing physical skills can have a great effect in the classroom and in her social interactions. It will also mean that the child might enjoy games lessons in future instead of dreading them.

If parents can afford it, and the child refuses to go to group classes because of feeling awkward, they could get a few private, one-to-one lessons that might make all the difference. (This worked with my daughter with her swimming lessons. She had trouble hearing what the instructor said when in a full class and she disliked the lessons. But after she'd had three one-to-ones at her local leisure centre, she realised she could swim well after all and this motivated her during the group classes, which she then enjoyed.)

If the child does go to group classes, parents could ask if she's made any friends, to show the expectation that she should talk to others: in the pool (when there is a break from instruction, while waiting for others to finish their swim or at the end if they have ten minutes' play) and in the changing room. It helps if the parent is seen by the child to talk to other parents in the changing room, as the parent is the child's role model: she needs to see the parent being friendly and outgoing. If the child does make a friend, she will enjoy the sessions much more. Other suggestions are:

- If the child is last to be picked for teams, could her teacher choose the groupings instead? Parents could try to find out if this is a problem for the child and, if it is, they could discuss it with the relevant teacher.

- If the child's ball skills are weak, parents could practise with her at home: catching, throwing, hitting with a racquet and kicking a ball.

- Can the child skip? For the unco-ordinated child, she may feel intensely embarrassed if all her friends in the schoolyard, for example, use a skipping rope and she can't. (Boys need to skip, too, for sports day and fitness training.) It is worthwhile for parents to find out what all the schoolyard fashions are so that the child is equipped with the relevant rope or yo-yo and is encouraged to practise at home.

Parents should never show disappointment that the child does not do well at sports and should never pressurise her with expectations before sports day. For some children, sports day is an experience of public humiliation and they look upon it with dread. Even if the child is last by a long chalk, parents should tell her it is important that she finishes the course so that she is applauded for sticking with it rather than giving up – for which she could expect to receive negative comments.

If sports day is an impending nightmare for the child, attendance should not be enforced. As with school trips, they are so rare that the child will not be desensitised by going to an annual event and there are probably much more pressing things to work on with the child that affect her daily life.

If the child is grossly overweight and is not good at sports for this reason, it is obviously a problem big enough to affect her physical as well as her mental health. She should be seen by her doctor for possible referral to a specialist. Children become more and more self-conscious as they get older, particularly when they hit puberty. Addressing a weight problem before this time would help the child's self-esteem and her physical health. However, any dieting should be prescribed by her doctor, and the child should not be made to feel bad about how she looks, as this can create other problems such as anorexia or bulimia nervosa.

Feeling an academic failure

Parents can:

- Ask the child's teacher to help if the child is struggling, to give ideas on how to help the child at home. This may alert the teacher to offering the child help in school, without always waiting for the child to ask specifically.

- Ask the child's teacher to be sensitive about asking the child to answer questions in front of the whole class or to read out loud. If this upsets the child, there is no reason why she should have to do this unless she volunteers. However, as with all social anxiety, the child should be continually challenged so that she pushes back the barriers of her anxiety. It would be good if she agreed to personal goals of trying to volunteer an answer a week, building up to an answer a day, until she is able to cope with the teacher giving her the odd question or two and reading out in class. But as long as she is trying to overcome her fears, definite goals should not be enforced, as the main aim is for the child to feel comfortable about being in school. If the child is continually working out of her area of security it will distress her, so she must be allowed to set the pace and be free not to move on to the second step until she is comfortable with the first, and so on.

- Increase the child's confidence by listening to her read every night so that her reading becomes more fluent. Parents can encourage the child to read with expression and can try taking parts at dramatic points to practise showing characters' feelings (also see *Becoming dramatic* later in the chapter).

- Get a tutor for the child (if parents can afford it and feel it's necessary) so that she can keep up with the rest of the class, or with the children on her table. This shouldn't, however, put unnecessary pressure on the child to perform well as this may have the opposite effect, lowering her self-confidence.

- Find out which maths and English books the school uses and buy them to help the child at home if the child's school won't let her take them out of school. Doing the work with the child, one to one, before she has to perform in class, will increase her confidence. She will then be relieved of the dread of having to do pages of corrections and being left behind by her peers. Also, if she is anxious, she will find it hard to take in her teacher's explanation of where she has gone wrong, being only worried about how soon she can be left to herself. If parents choose to do this, they should ensure they don't go too far ahead of the class with the child; the class teacher likes to keep children that sit at the same table in roughly the same place. For example, if a child finishes the required two pages quickly, she may then be directed to read to herself rather than continue with the maths and so race ahead of the others. Also, if the child is very far ahead of the others, there is a risk she will feel pressurised.

- Ask about the child's homework every night and get her to explain what she needs to do. Parents can help her where necessary and ensure that it is completed to the best of her ability. This does take time, but it gets the child into good habits so that eventually she will be able to direct herself and take responsibility for her own work.

- Help the child if she has to learn some lines to say in assembly or at a harvest festival service, for example, or in front of the class. Parents can check she is accurate, is easily understood, has introduced expression and can be easily heard – if not, the child can practise at the other end of the room and if her voice does not carry she can keep repeating the lines more loudly. Parents can demonstrate if necessary, although this may be beyond the capabilities of many very shy children. If the child is in a position to cope with it, she should be helped to do the best she can so that she feels proud of herself after the event and looks forward to having another opportunity to take part in something else. With social phobia, the child may be able to do some things and not others, so if she wants to give it a go, parents should encourage her.

Long-term school failure demoralises children and drastically lowers their self-esteem. It also distances the children from help that parents and teachers can give, making them disaffected with the education system. This can result in children dropping out of school early, not valuing qualifications and giving up trying to succeed. This in turn alienates children from peers who are academically successful and so they only feel akin to others who are also disaffected. These children might also exhibit anti-social tendencies such as shoplifting, joy-riding, drinking to excess and experimenting with illegal drugs, creating more problems. School needs to be viewed as a useful, friendly place by children for them to want to succeed academically.

Selective mutism

Selective mutism is a severe form of social phobia where children will not speak to anyone apart from very close friends and family (but not always everyone at home) in places where they feel relaxed. (It occurs in probably less than one per cent of children in elementary school settings.)[4, 5] It is dealt with in this book separately from social phobia, which has later onset (over age eight), because it starts in pre-school children; other social anxiety usually begins after the child has had a period of being comfortable in the school social environment. Also, selective mutism involves anxiety about speech, whereas later-onset social phobia is more wide ranging (although, of course, selectively mute children can have other anxieties too).

Selectively mute children would not, for example, be able to talk in school or at social events or in the company of individuals from outside the family when at home. It used to be called elective mutism, but that term is no longer used as it suggests that the child is being awkward and *choosing* not to speak, whereas, in reality she is so anxious she *cannot* speak.[4, 6] However, while face-to-face interaction would not be possible, some such children can talk on the telephone and many can be outgoing when at home.[7]

Selective mutism can develop in very young children and persist into adolescence, affecting their educational and social development; children who suffer from it usually need professional help. Selectively mute children have often shown shy and clingy behaviour as toddlers in the presence of people from outside the family, whereas they can talk and play normally when alone with close family members. The reluctance to speak becomes more noticeable when the child starts nursery or school, being in an environment where she is expected to speak.

The selectively mute child shows body language that indicates she is having to fight anxiety, such as making no eye contact, having a blank facial expression, being immobile (or having a frozen posture) or fidgeting nervously, when expected to contribute verbally in an insecure setting. Because the selectively mute child experiences great anxiety in social settings, there are often other anxiety disorders present as well (such as separation anxiety disorder, generalised anxiety disorder, panic disorder, PTSD and phobias).[5]

Selectively mute children communicate by nodding or shaking their heads, pointing, pulling and pushing, whispering, giving monosyllabic answers, talking in a monotone or by changing the sound of their voice.[7]

Onset of selective mutism

It has already been mentioned that children who develop selective mutism are a subset of inhibited children who have not learned to quiet their nervous reactions in social situations.[4] When they first became quiet, it is likely that family members helped them out by speaking for them, which enabled the situation to persist until the child only speaks to a few. Most selectively mute children have not experienced trauma.[5] More girls than boys seem to be affected by selective mutism, and young children have a higher incidence.[7]

It is thought that the combination of the child's temperament (being shy, a worrier, clingy, socially withdrawn and showing signs of social avoidance), together with a family history of anxiety behaviours (such as those mentioned in Chapter Two) and environmental change (such as having a new sibling, going to a new school or moving home) can lead to selective mutism.[8] Other possible contributory factors are having over-protective or domineering mothers or strict and remote fathers, having unresolved psychological conflict, trauma due to hospitalisation at a young age, or abuse. However, the condition is not fully understood because of a lack of research due to its relative rarity.[5]

Diagnosis of selective mutism

Children who suffer from selective mutism have a problem with anxiety. This is particularly true of some children who have autistic spectrum disorders, who are so anxious about speaking that they have trouble talking when stressed or stop talking altogether – but at other times they may talk incessantly about what interests them.

However, a professional may be needed to rule out other disorders to give a firm diagnosis. For example, if the onset of the child's mutism follows a head injury, that would have to be investigated rather than immediately attributing the lack of speech to selective mutism. Alternatively the child may have problems with speaking one language at home and being expected to converse in a different language at school (see below). Or the child may have a neurological disorder that has caused muscle weakness and co-ordination problems in her jaw, lips and tongue, or the child may have a problem with her hearing.

A diagnosis of selective mutism[9] is made when the child has avoided talking in certain situations for at least one month after the start of the school year, but does talk to family members in a home setting and understands what others say. The child's failure to speak is not due to a lack of knowledge of the spoken language, nor is it solely due to a communications disorder (such as stuttering), a psychotic disorder (such as schizophrenia) or a pervasive development disorder (such as autism and Asperger syndrome). The lack of verbal interaction must also put the child at a disadvantage educationally and socially for a diagnosis to be made. Early on in life, some children cope very well using gestures and sign language and so do not need to speak to get all they need from their environment, which may mean that help is not sought until the pattern has been well established.

If a child is learning one language at home and another in school, it is quite possible that she will feel uneasy about speaking in a strange language. This is not selective mutism from fear of speaking to people, but transient mutism, from not sufficiently knowing the language to communicate easily. Transient mutism soon passes as the child becomes more familiar with the new language. Another example of transient mutism is when a child suffers a trauma such as bereavement and then stops speaking altogether until the stress passes. Here the child might talk to no one at all, so it is not *selective* mutism.

Treatment of selective mutism

No one should pressure a selectively mute child to speak as this will worsen the condition and make the child more anxious. If a child shows selective mutism, she should be referred to a professional for behavioural therapy and, in some cases, medication: SSRI anti-depressants that increase the influence of serotonin in the brain leading to a reduction of anxious thoughts (see *Selective serotonin reuptake inhibitors* in Chapter Seven), as the combination of these can have a positive effect. The medication can be stopped when the child has started to speak in a variety of situations. Teaching the child relaxation techniques can also be beneficial and, if successful, may make medication unnecessary.[4] Reducing the child's anxiety is the first step in treatment, as the child will not speak if she remains desperately anxious in the social situation in which she is expected to speak.

The child then needs graduated exposure (starting with tiny steps to increase her verbal communication) so that she is desensitised to speaking in stressful situations. This approach is the same as for social phobia below, and as with social phobia, the programme of exposure will be individual to the child.

It also helps if the disorder is externalised by telling the child that her mutism stops her from having a good time and that she needs to fight against it. A record of graduated tasks can be kept, where the child tells the therapist whether it is she or the mutism that is winning, so as to help motivate the child and show her she can gain control.[4]

Selective mutism can last for a short time or persist for many years, where even as adults sufferers are struggling to speak in social environments. People need to understand that the child's silence is not intentional or wilful. Patience is needed to gain the child's trust – to encourage rather than force her to speak and to praise her whenever possible to make her feel more at ease.

One of the ways professionals help the selectively mute child is by role-playing social situations so that she becomes more confident and less worried about saying the wrong thing. They also look at the way the family operates to see if family members are unconsciously compounding the child's problems. The family joins therapy sessions, as they need to help the therapist. For example, the therapy might begin in the clinic without the therapist present to get the child used to playing and talking in a strange room. Through graduated exposure to the therapist, the child will be encouraged to speak in the clinic with the therapist present. Later, more situations will need to be introduced with the help of the family. (Also see *Positive behaviour changes: modelling* and *Desensitisation* in Chapter Seven.) Parents are encouraged to always show the child the expectation that she will speak and to encourage facial expressions and gestures as well.[10]

Improving the child's social confidence

A lack of social confidence can be related to a lack of academic prowess, physical prowess (both looked at earlier in the chapter), social prowess or a child's low self-esteem (these are looked at later in the chapter), making her believe that her performance is not up to scratch and will be negatively judged by others, even if this is not the case.

Helping to make the child more socially confident – in the way she holds herself (her body language), how she talks and in recognising the need to communicate effectively and be able to stand up for herself – will reduce her anxiety.

Improving the child's social competence

Social anxiety is related to how well a child feels she is performing socially compared to the people with whom she is interacting. Parents could help the child by:

- Regularly inviting friends round for the child to play with so that she closely bonds with them and feels at ease in their company. This helps her when she is at school, feeling protected and secure within her friendship group.

- Listening to the child's day at school to pick up on potential problems: early identification of bullying behaviour towards the child allows early intervention so that it can be stopped before it becomes a big problem, interfering with the child's willingness to attend school. Parents can pick up on other problems and discuss them with the child before they are blown out of proportion in her mind. An example of this is when she has been given homework but doesn't understand what she has to do and fears getting into trouble about it. A simple solution to this problem is for the child to ring up a friend and ask about it, or for parents to make the call. Failing this, a letter to her teacher may help, saying that the child was unable to do her homework because of not understanding what she had to do, and since her parents didn't know either, she couldn't be helped at home.

- Ensuring the child understands about good manners and basic social rules. For example, she can enhance her friendships by thanking friends for coming round, and seeing them to the door when it's time for them to go. It would be a mistake if she simply ignored them and carried on with a game alone, expecting them to find their own way out and not indicating that she found their company pleasurable.

- Doing a social skills training course with the child. A comprehensive book I wrote for parents and professionals to use with children aged 7 to 16 is *Social Awareness Skills for Children*: it is a text from which the whole family can gain.

- Practising difficult situations that are about to arise by role-playing them, so that the child has some idea of what to expect and how to behave, helps remove some of the fear of the unknown.

- Discussing with the child what she is worried about, if she can verbalise her fears, and then trying to allay her worries. If she's worried about saying something by mistake, for example, parents can tell her to say, 'I'm sorry, I didn't mean to say that. What I meant was...' Much difficulty children have is feeling that once something is said, they will be judged on it and they cannot retract or rephrase. Parents can show the child that this is not true in the way they speak to her. They can apologise for tactless or unfair things that are said and retell it how it should be, encouraging the child to do the same. ('That wasn't very nicely put. Would you like to have another try?')

- Learning about body language and passing on the knowledge to the child. (See *Confident body language* later in the chapter.) This will help her friendships and her dealings with teachers. For example, when a teacher asks her a question, the child should keep eye contact when she answers. It is rude to do otherwise. And her voice must be loud and clear enough to be understood and heard easily.

- Including the child as much as possible in all social aspects of the family. She could be encouraged, for example, to show off any new skill to Grandma so that she gets used to performing in front of others.

- Praising the child not only for what she does and says, but also for the times she instinctively knows to keep quiet, such as noticing when parents are telling a minor lie. Tact is a very hard skill to develop and through explaining the need for the lie, the child will gain a greater understanding of the complexities of social intercourse.

It is also important for the child to try to look confident even if she doesn't feel confident. This means sitting and standing straight rather than slumped with eyes glued to the floor. Looking confident helps the child to feel confident and others will recognise this and behave towards her in a more positive way. For example, if the child is asked a question in class and she looks embarrassed or squirms under the teacher's eye, she is more likely to receive sniggers from classmates as they see she is uncomfortable and ill at ease. Even if she cannot answer the question correctly, it doesn't matter. Others will perceive her differently just by the way she holds herself and projects her voice.

ASSERTIVENESS SKILLS

The child can become anxious if she feels out of control of a situation or feels that she is being forced to do something against her will, but doesn't have the courage to speak up. Parents and professionals can:

- Get the child to practise saying 'no' to people. She may find this impossible in school, even with friends, as she does not want to lose their approval. But it is important that she can do it. As well as it keeping her safe when someone suggests doing something silly, it regains control over part of her life that the child may feel is at everyone else's disposal. It helps to raise her self-esteem because she is considering her own needs and it shows her friends that they cannot ill-use her. When communicating with her teacher, she may have to refuse to do something while giving an explanation as to why. For example, if her teacher asks her to join the rest of the class in getting changed for games because she is lagging behind, she could say (when it is genuinely true), 'I'm sorry Miss, but I don't feel well.' Suffering in silence and not explaining why she doesn't want to do something just makes her feel more miserable. She has a right to stick up for her personal needs and get others to recognise them.

- Explain to the child the rights all children have (reproduced from page 103 of my book, *Social Awareness Skills for Children*):

  o I have the right to say what I need.

  o I have the right to say what things are important to me.

  o I have the right to do well without worrying about others being jealous of me.

  o I have the right to refuse (that is, to say 'no').

  o I have the right to ask for help when I need it.

  o I have the right to ask for more time to think when I have to make an important decision.

  o I have the right to say, 'I don't know' without others making me feel silly.

  o I have the right to say, 'I don't understand' without others making me feel small.

  o I have the right to make up my own mind about things.

  o I have the right to change myself.

- o I have the right to make mistakes (as long as they're not done on purpose).

- o I have the right to move on from past mistakes without everyone reminding me of them.

The child can make a poster for her wall with these rights listed in bold and bright colours, and become used to mentioning the rights with other members of the family. If parents remind the child of their own rights, she should start reminding them of hers and then she will take this confidence into her own social group. (She doesn't have to tell her friends about each right they have violated, but simply use the knowledge that such a violation occurred and point out the unfairness. It should soon stop unjust behaviour towards her or unjust expectations of her.)

CONFIDENT BODY LANGUAGE

Body language is about the way the child's body looks and how her voice sounds and how closely she stands to the next person. Most of anyone's communication is through body language: only a tiny percentage of information is passed through the actual words spoken. Other children and adults can see in a moment if the child looks uncomfortable or shy and, depending on their perspective, they may either try to make a special effort to help her or take advantage of her obvious lack of confidence.

In teaching the child confident body language, she is more protected (as long as she can make use of it in a convincing way) against bullying, and against adults and other children poking fun. They are far more likely to take the child seriously and not assume that, for example, because she is so shy they will be able to get away with manipulative or unfair behaviour. Confident body language includes:

- Standing, or sitting up, straight.

- Facing the person the child is talking or listening to, squarely.

- Making eye contact with the other person.

- Speaking with a firm, clear voice at a volume loud enough to be heard easily, but not a shout.

- Sounding confident about the opinions or answers the child gives. If the child is saying 'no', she should sound as though she expects others to accept this without question, otherwise they will see it as an invitation to persuade her to change her mind. She should also pronounce the word firmly, without mumbling.

Improving the child's self-esteem

Social anxiety is also related to how the child views herself. A confident child may have a high self-esteem and therefore assume that other people want to know her and be friends with her. This will make her socially confident and socially successful. However, a shy, unconfident child will have negative thoughts relating to social contact with others (although in young children, they may only be conscious of feeling uncomfortable rather than having specific negative thoughts) and this will hamper her spontaneity and eagerness to meet and interact with others.

The following will help raise the child's self-esteem and can be used with any child, not just the shy, unconfident ones:

- The child could think of everything she can do, everything she is good at and everything nice anyone has ever said about her and write them down. She can have the list on her wall or in a prominent place to remind her of all her achievements and all her good qualities: from being kind to her cat to skilfully kicking a ball around, to being brave about visits to the dentist.

- Parents should frequently tell the child that they love her and always will (and when necessary, also tell her that this is not dependent on her doing well at things: it is unconditional love).

- The child should be told that she is special. She is completely unique. There is no one else in the world quite like her. There is only one … (the child's name).

- The child should be praised whenever possible to make her feel good about herself and protect her from being damaged by ridicule, and she should be told what characteristics people like about her (such as her sense of fun). She should only be praised when it is deserved, otherwise it becomes meaningless and the child will doubt the value of what people say even when it is genuine.

- Parents should tell the child how proud they are of her for being so brave when she's frightened.

- The child should be told that many things just don't matter and that they will sort themselves out, such as children developing different skills at different rates. If she is behind in one thing, she is probably ahead in another.

- What the child wears is very important to her. Parents should ensure that she is seen to be wearing fashionable clothes and shoes that fit. (This is not prescribing expensive 'designer' clothes.)

- The child should be gently questioned about her friends and others in her class to identify bullying behaviour, of either the child or another child. This helps the child's awareness of bullying behaviour, and what to do about it can then be discussed. (Ideas are given in Chapter Three: Bullying.)

- The child should not be negatively judged in her hearing. If she hears people being critical of her, she will assume that others will see the same shortcomings and come to the same conclusion so will fear having to repeat the thing in company, such as a wobbly handstand.

- Parents should not hint by word or deed that they are in any way disappointed with the child, unless it is over something small that they genuinely feel she could have managed but chose not to. (This may be difficult because these problems are very subjective and parents will need to know the child intimately to judge this.)

- The child should be spoken to as an equal, valuing her opinion and seeking her advice over things with which she could help.

- The child should not be blamed for anything that is not her fault; personal frustration and anger should not be taken out on her. (And, if it is, the child deserves an apology.)

- Adults should listen to how they interact with the child. Is the majority of feedback she gets from them positive or do they nag unnecessarily or show their disappointment by sighing or being sarcastic with her? If so, they should try to be more gentle, understanding and tolerant.

- The child should never be put down: if she does something wrong, she'll probably know it without adults having to say something like, 'Typical!' This is a particularly non-useful comment as it describes the child generally, labelling her in a negative way. If adults want to chastise, they could say something like, 'That was a silly thing to do, don't you think?' (This does not label the child, but her behaviour.) A sensitive child needs careful middle-ground handling, where she is not allowed to get away with bad behaviour but to have it acknowledged that, when an accident occurs, that's just what it is and she should not be labelled as clumsy, for example.

- If the child does something out of character, she should be asked why she did it instead of brushing it aside or telling her off. It might give adults insight into the way her mind works and it may be that they'd totally misread the situation. This will help her trust adults more.

- The child's feelings should not be disregarded. If she's upset, she shouldn't be told to pull herself together and act her age. The matter should be gently discussed and a solution sought with the child's help. This helps her gain the confidence to work out similar problems on her own when she's older. Everyone, however, throughout life, comes across new situations that they don't know how to handle, so it would be unrealistic to think that this is a one-off training that lasts for life. But what it does do is teach her that if she can't solve a problem on her own, to go and find someone who can help.

- Parents should have fun with the child on a regular basis or the child might see life with them as very functional and matter-of-fact, which might make the child feel out of touch with them. To be emotionally close, special moments need to be shared.

- Parents should give the child as much responsibility as she can handle. They could let her choose what she eats, for example, when choice is convenient to them, so that she directs some of her life and does not feel totally controlled; but food should not be used as either punishment or reward – it should be a neutral thing. (However, it is okay to say she can have her chocolate bar, for example, when she has had an apple or that she must have some fruit after the chocolate.) The child could choose the order in which she does things, such when to shower, when to do her homework and which television programmes she wants to watch (if parents limit her viewing and expect her to be selective). Parents should also let the child help in the home such as by taking responsibility for looking after a pet or by posting letters. The tasks should be pleasant so that she will mostly enjoy doing them and be pleased about her extra responsibility without feeling used. Parents should always thank her for her help.

SELF-CONFIDENCE

This is related to how the child feels about herself, without having to rely on positive comments from others for her to believe she's doing well. And it is not feeling a need to compare herself with others before she can feel proud of her achievements; it is measuring herself against how she was and how she's doing now.

If the child sets herself impossible goals (or she feels her parents have), she will worry about not being able to fulfil them and will consider herself a failure if she can't. Lowering goals, without giving up trying alltogether, is a sensible compromise. No one can be perfect and no one should expect to be.

True self-confidence is an inner acceptance of who the child feels she is, and is seen in the positive way in which she can relate to others.

THE CHILD'S APPEARANCE

Many younger children like to look the same as everyone else (helped by school uniform) by wearing the same type of clothes from the same shops as the majority, and similar shoes. They do not like to stand out as different in any way: they prefer to merge with the crowd. Parents should try to ensure that the child feels comfortable with what she wears as it will give her confidence to feel part of a group.

They should also ensure that she is clean and neat, at least on arrival at school. Children avoid 'smelly' children and prefer to be with others who look smart. When they are adolescents they may play down the 'smart', but popular children still tend to be well presented (clean and brushed hair, clean face and hands, clean and ironed clothes).

When children hit adolescence they often like to be seen as individuals and so will not necessarily follow the same dress code as their peers. They may take steps to look different, even when wearing school uniform. (They might do this by wearing their tie to one side or rolling up their sleeves, or by rolling down their socks or wearing their sweatshirt tied about their waist.) But usually, these are more rebellious children and so may be less likely to suffer social anxiety, as they are happy to be more adventurous and defy convention in the search for their own identity. However, all adolescents are vulnerable at a time of bodily change and new awareness of themselves while under the critical eye of others, so the possibility of the child suffering from social anxiety must not be discounted: sometimes, the reason for an adolescent to rebel is the very fact that she doesn't feel comfortable with people and so pretends disinterest.

DYSMORPHOPHOBIA

Dysmorphophobia is a fear of body defects. Although this is not social phobia, it does interfere with the sufferer's social interactions, making her want to avoid meeting people. Having a poor body image gives a child a very low self-esteem. The child's anxiety is not just present during social interactions as with social phobia – it is there all the time. Social phobics know that what they feel and think is illogical, but children with dysmorphophobia do not. They take it very seriously indeed. The defect may be trivial to others (or even seem imaginary), yet is considered to be very noticeable by the sufferer and can dominate her life.

Dysmorphophobia usually starts in adolescence or early adulthood, when the person is very aware of her body and bodily changes that have taken or are taking place. Often the child feels that part of her is too large or too small, misshapen or that a region of her body smells. No matter how often the child is reassured, she will not be convinced that her body is okay, and will take extreme measures to hide whatever part she doesn't like with make-up, clothes or perfume. If the child has dysmorphophobia, she needs professional help.

Dealing with shyness and making new friends

Shyness can be a huge problem for many children, and some don't grow out of it, although it may become less intense. Shy children can be helped by learning how to behave and being given possible conversation starters by parents before each social occasion.

Usually, children are only shy when they do not feel confident. For example, a shy child is not usually shy with her own family; she can be as loud and argumentative as anyone else. It is when she is in situations where she does not feel at ease that the shyness kicks in. So the way forward is to help the child be more and more comfortable in more social situations: she needs more practice than non-shy children.

For example, if the child is going somewhere new, perhaps joining a club where she does not know any of the other children, parents could suggest ways for her to make friends quickly such as by using some of the following conversation starters:

- 'What's your name?'

- 'How long have you been coming here?'

- 'Where do you live?'

- 'What school do you go to?'

- 'Have you got brothers and sisters?'
- 'Do you have pets?'
- 'How old are you?'
- 'What year are you in?'

If the child were to use all these questions one after the other, she would sound like an interrogator. Ideally, the child she asks the first question to will answer and then ask the same question back. It may be that he then asks one of his own. However, if the other child is not so hot on social skills either so that he doesn't ask the same question back or a similar one, the child can volunteer information at the same level, matching the information she receives. This helps to make the new relationship balanced.

Giving information at the same level means not going into greater depth. For example, if the child asks another if he has brothers and sisters and he answers that he has one sister younger than him, but no brother, the child should give similar information, such as how many siblings she has and possibly their ages. But it would be inappropriate to give further details to a complete stranger, for example that her brother was adopted and is HIV positive and her teenage sister is having a baby. The child needs to know the difference between general information and private information that she should only reveal to a trusted few.

It is usually easier for a child to make a new friend with someone of the same sex and similar age because it usually requires more confidence to chat to older children (who may not want to be seen associating with a much younger child) and to members of the opposite sex. However, age is not always easy to judge, as some children are much taller than one would expect for their age and others are much shorter.

Sadly, not all children can be friends together regardless of age, as many children seem to set store on status: being seen with the right people, wearing the right clothes and doing the right sort of thing, whereas adult relationships are far more diverse and friendships can easily span a generation. Children, unfortunately, often lack the maturity and confidence to move away from expected behaviour, and because none of their friends may include younger children, they may not want to either.

Explaining all aspects of social life to the child will reduce the number of mistakes she makes and she can more easily understand how the social world functions, rather than being confused by the whole thing and feeling a failure, taking rejection personally, when it has nothing whatever to do with herself as a person.

As well as understanding social dynamics, addressing the thoughts the child has that interfere with her ability to make relaxed social contact can help shyness. For example, sometimes a child's self-esteem may be so low she cannot imagine anyone wanting to be friends with her. If parents think this might be so with the child, they could ask her what thoughts stop her from initiating conversation with her peers and other people she meets. They could then write them down and with the child try to think of alternative, realistic thoughts, although many children struggle to cope with challenging negative thoughts so not all will pick up this technique easily.

EXAMPLE

1. No one will want to talk to me because I have nothing interesting to say.

    Alternative thought: I don't need to have something to say to talk to someone. I can ask about the other person instead. People love to talk about themselves.

2. I'm boring.

    Alternative thought: If I stop thinking about how uninteresting and boring I am, concentrate on the actual event and have some things ready to talk about, I'll be fine. Even if I think I'm boring, there is no reason why others will know this is how I feel.

3. I don't know what to say because I don't know what the other person is interested in.

    Alternative thought: If I listen to other people's conversations, I can tell that they aren't worrying about whether the other person is interested – they often talk about what interests them. If I do the same, I'll soon know whether the other person is interested because he'll ask questions if he is and look bored if he isn't. He might volunteer something that he wants to say. It might be just the right topic and then there'll be no problem. We can't guess what interests others; we have to find out by trial and error, by volunteering information and asking questions. And someone has to start the ball rolling. It may as well be me.

4.   People don't like me.

Alternative thought: That can't apply to everyone. I must work out how to justify this statement. Can I prove that they don't? What evidence is there for it? Should I base my entire judgement on one short meeting? And, if I really think they don't like me, why is that? Is it because I don't look pleased to see them and show interest in them? Perhaps if I change my approach, they will change theirs.

5.   I'm too shy to make the first move.

Alternative thought: Am I really too shy or can't I be bothered to make the effort? As I get older I become more and more of an adult and an excuse like shyness becomes less valid. By allowing myself to hide behind my shyness I am preventing others from getting to know the real me. Also, to others it would seem like I am disinterested and rude if I don't make an effort. They don't know me so they won't know I'm shy.

Dealing with loneliness

A child who lacks social skills can become lonely because others do not find her company rewarding. All social interactions are two-way, with both sides gaining something from the relationship at some time, even if not every time they meet. For example, mutually rewarding company is when people can laugh together, have fun, share similar interests and topics of conversation, and do things together.

It can also be rewarding when one person listens to someone else's problems and manages to comfort him or offer suggestions on what to do. If a child is able to help out a friend in need by listening to his problems, she rewards him by taking his problems seriously and by giving sympathy and understanding. The child herself is also rewarded: by being able to offer help and by feeling pleased that the friend chose to unburden himself to her.

However, if the relationship is continually one-sided, with one child always having to give while the other expects to take with no return, the friendship may fail. Rewarding behaviour can include:

- Showing sensitivity towards others.

- Looking pleased to see other people by smiling and greeting them in a cheerful way.

- Sharing jokes and funny experiences.

- Listening to what others have to say without interrupting.

- Noticing when someone looks sad and asking him what the matter is.

- Showing care when things go wrong for others.

An absolute no-no is making fun of other people or taking advantage of bad things that happen to them, such as laughing when someone drops her PE kit in the toilet by mistake. (It is only all right to laugh when something like this happens if the person involved laughs too.)

Unfortunately, a lonely child can pick up on messages received about others not wanting her company and may believe that there is no point in trying to make new friends because no one would want to know her anyway. This is a vicious circle that must be broken. The child cannot write off all other children because of a few negative experiences. Adults should try to discuss what went wrong in those relationships and how they can be rescued, or how the child can ensure that the same thing doesn't happen again.

Social phobia in older children

This section applies to older children, aged about 14 upward, who have social phobia or social anxiety.

Social phobics may be perceived as aloof, awkward, backward, disinterested, inhibited, nervous, quiet, shy, unfriendly and withdrawn despite their wanting to make friends and become involved, being hampered by their anxiety. Although they know the fear and panic they experience is illogical, they cannot change their negative thoughts or reduce their anxiety without professional help. Some of the fears social phobics have are:

- Fear of being the centre of attention.

- Fear of being watched or observed while doing something and having others notice, for example, how their hands shake (such as when pouring a drink or signing a document) or voices shake (such as when making telephone calls). The fear creates sufficient tension for these things to happen and so sufferers feel they are failures and fear the situation all the more the next time.

- Fear of being teased or criticised. In anxiety, sufferers may not realise they are being teased, take other people's comments literally and so give inappropriate responses and are then embarrassed when everyone laughs or they may take the criticism to heart and reply in a heavy-handed way, making them seem churlish. These can give them negative experiences that make them dread similar situations, feeling they are the butt of everyone's jokes and that others are just waiting for them to make the next mistake so they can have another good laugh.

- Fear of humiliation; for example, of tripping up, knocking things over, saying the wrong things, spilling food or drink, or of no one wanting to talk to them.

- Fear of being introduced to other people. They may not be able to remember other people's names or be able to think of anything to say.

- Fear of having to say something in a formal, public situation.

- Fear of having to meet and talk to people in authority. The stakes are perceived as being higher here and they feel more pressurised to 'succeed'.

- Fear of vomiting. Anxiety about the social situation can cause nausea, making them worry about being sick, causing more worry, which can eventually make them vomit. If the fear about vomiting is ever present – such as when they're with people who have been drinking alcohol or declare they're getting over a flu bug – and they worry unreasonably about catching it, then they are probably also emetophobic (emetophobics fear being sick themselves and being present when others vomit).

- Fear of fainting. Anxiety can make them feel faint although fainting is unlikely, as anxiety raises blood pressure.

- Fear of choking on food, of not being able to swallow or of spilling food down themselves. Anxiety can constrict their throat muscles, making swallowing feel very uncomfortable, and it can make their movements shaky and jerky, increasing the likelihood of spilling something.

- Fear of having diarrhoea (anxiety can cause this).

- Fear of blushing and others noticing it.

- Fear of having to shake hands, knowing theirs are sweaty from anxiety and that anyone they shake hands with will want to wipe them afterwards.

Some children worry about needing the toilet when with others or that others may notice how often they go (anxiety increases the need to urinate and defecate), or that they will need to go desperately when no toilet is available and risk humiliating themselves by not being able to 'hold on'. Others are anxious about going to the toilet with others nearby and may not be able to 'go' until they are completely alone, being unable to use public toilets, for example. These anxieties are known as sphincteric phobias and revolve around social situations.

Treatment of social phobia

Professionals use cognitive behavioural therapy (see Chapter Seven) to treat social phobia. The cognitive part is finding alternative, helpful thoughts to use to counteract children's negative thoughts (as shown above). The behavioural part is desensitising the sufferer to her anxiety through gradually increasing exposure to fearful situations (see below).

If untreated, social phobia can pervade every aspect of the child's life so that she finds it hard to interact with others at all.

The way to desensitise anyone with social phobia is to first of all consider all the social things that the sufferer can do without anxiety, what she can do with some anxiety and what she feels is totally beyond her. Each desensitisation programme is individual to the person.

For example, for someone who enjoys talking to others one-to-one and can drink in other people's company but cannot eat with anyone else, feels uncomfortable in other people's homes (feeling the need to escape), and has trouble making new friends, one could draw up the following programme in ascending order of difficulty:

1. Maintain the social contacts I already have so that I don't lose confidence about doing those things.

2. Try to interact with people I meet when I'm out of the home, such as saying 'hello' to a neighbour or smiling at someone as I pass him or her. (This can give me confidence as the experience can bring the reward of someone smiling back or of exchanging pleasantries on a zero-commitment level.)

3. Arrange for friends to visit me at home.

4. Visit friends in their homes.

5. Meet a friend to go shopping with (to increase trust and familiarity so that when an opportunity comes later to eat with him or her, it is easier).

6. Meet a friend to go to the theatre or cinema with (escape is harder here because I am expected to remain for the length of the performance).

7. Practise eating with members of my family present:

   (a) Eat an apple or pot of yoghurt in the same room as other family members while everyone is watching television so that their attention isn't focused on me.

   (b) I could extend this to bags of crisps and biscuits and other TV snacks. (Dry food is harder to eat when I'm anxious because my saliva dries up.)

(c) I could eat a cold meal with others while watching television, such as sandwiches that are passed round to everyone that I can accept or decline, or they can be laid on a table so we can help ourselves.

(d) I could eat a meal, such as breakfast, in the kitchen, at the table with my family.

(e) I could eat a main meal with my family.

8. Eat every meal with my family.

9. Eat a meal with my family and a guest such as my brother's friend or my grandpa.

10. Increase the number of people with whom I eat while at home.

11. Eat my packed lunch with friends in school.

12. Meet a friend to have a drink with in a public place.

13. Go to a buffet party where no one will notice whether I eat much, if at all.

14. Invite someone for a drink and some cake at my home.

15. Accept food at a friend's home.

16. Make a new friend by inviting someone back to my home or suggesting that we meet for a drink.

17. Invite someone for a meal.

18. Invite several people for a meal.

19. Accept invitations to dine at other people's homes.

20. Accept invitations to have a take-away at other people's homes.

21. Accept invitations to dine out in a restaurant.

For social phobics who have anxiety involving eating or drinking with other people, it is important that no comment or criticism is made about how little they eat or drink in company. Asking them if they are anorexic, for example, is not likely to help. Sufferers want to eat and drink but anxiety makes it hard or even impossible for them to do this in company. Only when the focus is off them do they have a chance to relax sufficiently to do these things. A second example is for someone who does not like any attention focused on her in school:

1. Attend school.

2. Talk to all the people I usually talk to and smile at them.

3. Smile at two other schoolmates and talk to someone new.

4. Smile at teachers as I pass them in corridors.

5. Say 'hello' to the teachers I know well as I pass them in corridors.

6. Ask a teacher a question, in private at the end of the lesson.

7. Talk to the same teacher in front of other schoolmates.

8. Offer to help when a teacher asks for volunteers.

9. Offer to answer a question when a teacher addresses the whole class.

10. Volunteer to read aloud in front of the rest of the class.

11. Accept a small role in assembly.

12. Accept a small role in the school performance (or offer to hand out programmes on the night, or help backstage).

13. Do more of the above in more situations.

The steps in the above programmes should be carried out at each stage as often as possible, with the sufferer only going down the list once the things before have been mastered, so that she is not overwhelmed with anxiety, but can gradually push back her personal barriers. Once the anxiety of doing one thing is low enough to be tolerated, the sufferer should try to move on to the following step and, in this way, steps that are far behind become much easier and may no longer produce any anxiety symptoms at all.

Trying to proceed too quickly can dash the child's confidence and make her not want to try further, believing that she is getting worse via the programme instead of better. Also, she may occasionally need some time off. For example, if she is getting over flu, she may remember feeling sick and weak and worry that she will continue to feel like this when in a stressful environment, not having the mental strength to overcome her fears at this time. With such setbacks, the sufferer may need to start again with easier stages, but because of increased confidence, her progress to the stage she'd achieved previously should be quicker once her health is fully recovered and her daily occupation is resumed. However, long gaps should not grow between doing things that have been mastered or she may lose confidence again.

Although it is tempting for the sufferer to avoid situations that cause her panic, this will only make things worse. She does need to desensitise herself gradually to stressful situations in order to overcome social anxiety. And she should try, every time, to see social interactions as an opportunity to get to know others more deeply and to enjoy herself. Other things that can help a social phobic child increase her confidence are:

1.   using confident body language (introduced earlier in this chapter: below it is considered whether the child can make use of what she has learnt)

2.   using relaxation techniques

3.   using assertiveness skills

4.   getting fit and strong

5.   becoming dramatic

6.   changing the negative thoughts she has.

These are dealt with in order below.

USING CONFIDENT BODY LANGUAGE

Can the child look confident when she is asked to? She needs to be able to behave in a confident way even when she is anxious. This is for two reasons:

1.   If she looks confident and behaves in a confident manner, she is more likely to feel confident. Teachers know all about this. Even when they dread a particular class, they know that they must look and behave in a confident way in order to fulfil pupils' expectations of teachers and not let them think they have someone of whom they can take advantage.

2. It is her form of protection. Part of social phobia is worrying that people will guess how nervous the sufferer is. Even if she is nervous, as long as others can't guess it, she's got away with it and they'll not think her any different to the next person.

The sufferer should practise sitting, standing and walking confidently at home. She should also practise speaking confidently while looking people squarely in the eye. (She can practise talking in front of the mirror.) The more she practises it, the more likely that confident behaviour will become second nature to her. By behaving confidently, she will command more respect and have a 'presence', and she will notice how others respond to this. Confident body language could be made into a game where everyone in the household has to behave in a confident manner (even when saying 'sorry').

If parents have a video camera, taking shots of the child before and after her confident body language training will help her feel proud of her achievement. And seeing herself as she is when she behaves unconfidently will help her understand what she has to put right.

The training could be tested by asking the child to walk into a newsagents to buy a magazine, to smile at everyone she passes in the shop and at the assistant who takes her money. She can say, 'Hello, I'd like to buy this' as she hands it over, smiling. If the assistant bothers to make eye contact with her, the child is likely to get a smile back and perhaps a comment. But if she approaches the counter in silence and hands over the money without making eye contact, the assistant is almost guaranteed not to take any notice of her either. When the child leaves, she should say 'thanks' for any change and then 'goodbye'.

This game could be made into a challenge. How many strangers can the child get to notice her in shops (or in other safe environments where her friendliness won't be misinterpreted)? And which does she prefer? Being invisible and ignored by everyone or being noticed as a friendly and outgoing person?

Using confident body language is not an exercise to do and then forget about. It needs constant practice and should become part of the child's life. Everyone has times when things go wrong and they want the ground to swallow them up. It's okay to feel like that, but not to look it. It's okay for her to say 'sorry', she's made a terrible mistake or tell a friend about what has happened. But she still needs to hold herself erect and not let the situation make her feel so low that she shows the whole world how she feels. Being able to do this will give her enormous inner strength.

USING RELAXATION TECHNIQUES

Although young children cannot be taught how to relax, teenagers can (although if the person has an autistic spectrum disorder this can make her more anxious).[11] It is also possible for children aged eight or nine and above to learn with help. Even if they cannot remember everything when in a state of panic, they may still be able to use relaxation to calm them before sleep using a relaxation cassette or CD (see suggestions in *Further Resources*). There are three things to consider in teaching relaxation:

1. The child's breathing
When a child is anxious, she does not breathe using her diaphragm. If anxiety has continued over a long period she may have stopped breathing like this altogether, except when asleep. The importance of breathing using the diaphragm is that chest-breathing leads to hyperventilation, which will make her feel ill, worsening her anxiety.

When the child is sitting or lying down, she should be asked to put one hand on her chest and one on her abdomen. Breathing in through her nose and out through her mouth, her chest should not move, but her abdomen should (she can push it out as she breathes in). Breathing in through the nose helps her to stop hyperventilating as nostrils are smaller than the mouth so it takes longer for the breath to fill her lungs. And breathing out through the mouth means that she has to concentrate on what she is doing, so it distracts her panicking mind: it can be a releasing experience, letting go all her tension at the same time.

In order for this to be used as a calming method, diaphragmatic breathing needs to be practised until it is almost second nature. Relaxation cassettes or CDs can teach her how to do this. (See *Further Resources*.)

For general calming, a small dot of Tippex (correction fluid) could be put on the face of the child's watch. Every time she looks at her watch, she will see this dot and it will remind her to check her breathing and modify it by breathing diaphragmatically and in through her nose. Doing this numerous times a day brings down her overall stress levels and reduces the severity of the physical symptoms caused by hyperventilation (such as faintness and nausea).

There is another breathing technique that is calming, taught to me in a yoga class many years ago. If the child is panicky, she can go to another room to be alone or to the toilet. There she can spend ten minutes carrying out the following instructions:

(a) Using your right hand place your thumb over your right nostril and your third finger over your left nostril.

(b) Let your first and second fingers rest gently on the bridge of your nose.

(c) Close your left nostril and breathe out through your right nostril.

(d) Breathe in through the same nostril and close your thumb over it.

(e) Count to three while holding your breath.

(f) Breathe out through your left nostril, releasing the pressure of your third finger.

(g) Breathe in again through the same nostril, then close it.

(h) Hold your breath and count to three.

(i) Release your right nostril and breathe out.

(j) Breathe in again through the same nostril and close it.

(k) Hold your breath and count to three...and so on.

In other words, throughout the exercise the breath must escape through the opposite nostril to that through which the breath was taken in. This is an excellent calming method as it stops hyperventilation and, because it requires much concentration to do it properly, it also distracts the mind.

Once learnt, this exercise can be added to. As the child breathes in, she can imagine following the air flowing through her nostril, past her throat, down her windpipe and into her lungs, and when she holds her breath she can imagine the oxygen being taken from her lungs around her body by the bloodstream while carbon dioxide is dumped into her lungs. And when the child breathes out, she can imagine following the used air up her windpipe, past her throat and out through her nostril. This is so demanding on her concentration that it will, if done correctly, give her a complete break from panicky thoughts that might help turn the tide when she stops the exercise.

2. The child's muscle tension

A stressed child will have tense muscles, very often in the head, neck and abdomen. Relaxation cassettes and CDs (see *Further Resources* for suggestions) that systematically instruct the listener to tense, hold and then relax muscle groups could help relieve her muscle tension. The child can then experience a state of total relaxation and later remember what it feels like. Doing this every night at bedtime will help her get to sleep, help her stay asleep without early waking, and give her better quality sleep. She can also follow a cassette or CD in the daytime too if she feels anxious. Parents may want to do the exercise with her for the first couple of times so that she has company, feels less silly about doing it and so that parents share the experience.

As with the previous suggestion, if the child has a white dot on her watch, she can check her muscle tension when she checks her breathing. If her muscles feel tense, she can tense all of them, hold to a slow count of three and then release them to achieve a more relaxed state or, if in company, she can mentally tell herself to relax while imagining warm water trickling down her, giving her inner peace.

3. The child's thoughts

Negative thoughts will just increase the child's tension and may lead to panic. She must mentally tell herself to STOP and replace them with helpful thoughts. If these helpful thoughts are prepared beforehand, she can repeat them like a mantra: 'I've done this loads of times before. Although it's hard I know I can do it again.'

If the child is building up to a panic, she shouldn't try to fight it: she must try to let the feelings wash over her. It is only by ignoring them that they will lose their power. If necessary, she should distract herself with whatever is to hand. She could, for example, closely examine a pen: how it looks, how it feels to touch, its weight, its nib, its switch, its curves and its level of ink (if visible). Or she could start to count the number of bricks in a wall: how many in each row and how many rows.

It is inevitable that the child, once used to panic attacks, will have them recur. If she accepts that this will happen and neither sees them as failure nor tries to fight them, they should reduce in intensity. The less importance she attaches to them, the less power they will have over her. Eventually, she will recognise early warning signs of stress so that she can deflect her panic through positive ('I can beat this') or helpful ('I know what it's all about so it's not going to freak me out') thoughts or distraction. The key to overcoming her fear is to concentrate, not on herself, but on the people and things around her.

It is inevitable that a child will feel low after a panic attack, seeing it as a kind of failure. She can have another mantra for these times: 'Having trouble in this area of my life does not label me a failure. I am special and lovable. There is only one me and I am unique.'

USING ASSERTIVENESS SKILLS

Assertiveness is not about being aggressive or passive, but a middle ground where respect for the other person is always maintained unless that person has definitely done something to deserve a non-assertive (aggressive) response. The assertive child will check first whether there is an explanation for the other's behaviour before acting. (Also see *Assertiveness skills* earlier in the chapter.)

As well as respecting others, being assertive is about the child demanding respect for herself in the most appropriate way. She can do this by not letting others take advantage of her (she must learn to say 'no' at times), not letting others put her down and not letting injustices go without pointing them out.

If her awareness of prejudicial and stereotypical comments is raised, such as with racist and sexist remarks that are often used as put-downs, as are comments on people's appearance, accent or perceived sexuality, she will be better prepared to deal with them: 'That's wrong. Actually, …' or 'I think you've been misinformed…' In responding to put-downs, she should not start the sentence with 'You …' as the other person can perceive this as aggressive and confrontational. It is better to say, 'I think that…' or 'I don't agree with you because…'

A skilful communicator can also negotiate to find common ground with someone to reach a satisfactory compromise so that both sides 'win'. Not always being the 'loser' will raise the child's self-esteem and confidence.

To learn more about assertiveness skills, parents and professionals could do a social skills training course with the child (I've written books to help in this area: *People Skills for Young Adults* and *The People Skills Bible*) or by following an assertiveness course (as in my book, *Assertiveness For Young Adults*). All are suitable for young people aged 15 to 16 plus, the first being particularly suited to young people with mild learning difficulties.

Gloria Gaynor's song, *I Am What I Am* is about being assertive and demanding self-respect and respect from others ('I am what I am, and what I am needs no excuses...'). This song emphasises personal acceptance and getting the world to accept the individual too. Much strife stems from wanting to be something the child is not and from comparing herself unfavourably with others. The child can listen to the words of this song and incorporate them into her life (see *Further Resources*).

GETTING FIT AND STRONG

Being physically fit increases stamina and makes the child feel good about herself. Physical exercise also reduces stress and can help her sleep. If the child is physically well, with no reason not to exercise, she should be encouraged to get involved in sports. She may feel a failure in the rest of her life, so this might be something where she feels she can succeed. An anxious child may spend inordinate amounts of time at home with parents without getting the exercise her body needs.

It helps if there are things the family can do together that the child will enjoy and find non-threatening, such as running around the garden kicking a ball or hitting it with a racquet or playing catch, or going for walks and runs in the park, or going swimming. The family or a neighbour might have a dog that needs to be exercised regularly.

If the child is anxious about going outside the home, perhaps she can be given jobs to do around the home to make her feel useful. Fetching and carrying up and down stairs (if the home has them) is a good form of exercise.

The child should also be encouraged to dance to music. She can experiment moving her body to all types of music: pop songs, classical music, rock 'n' roll… There might be a friend with whom she'd like to make up a dance routine. Dancing is important for teenagers of both sexes, as much socialising takes place at discos.

BECOMING DRAMATIC

Parents can read aloud with the child from exciting parts of a book, or pretend to be newscasters. Parents can experiment with different roles and voices in reading, taking parts and exaggerating some of the characters' mannerisms, or copying eccentric famous people or an eccentric relative. This may help the child become more outgoing by making her more confident in roles where she would, in public, feel ridiculous. It is fine to be silly and have fun and, when there is no one else around to see, she can nurture a talent for mimicking, trying out regional accents, exhibiting body language that fits the characters she is reading about and be better able to express herself.

For example, many social phobics are socially withdrawn and do not like to be loud or show their feelings in public. But if the child has read out the part of an anguished mother, she learns how to express feelings in her voice, which she can use when she feels like that herself. The child could also play the part of someone very angry: it will help stop her from continually suppressing her own feelings.

Another useful piece of drama is for parent and child to swap roles. The parent can be the younger child while the child is the parent. She must look after her parent and keep him or her from harm (the age and skill level of this 'younger child' can be varied). Instead of just taking something dangerous out of the younger child's hand, for example, she must tell the younger child that he or she mustn't pick up knives and why they can be dangerous. She must also chastise when necessary (the younger child can be deliberately naughty, trying the child's patience) and even get angry. She must also comfort the younger child when he or she is in distress. Swapping roles may make the child feel, for a while, more confident and in control and personally powerful. If the child can do this with her parent, she could try talking to a real younger child who needs help.

As the child grows in confidence from role-playing, she should try to store in her memory how it feels to be confident and how she stands when she is.

It would be beneficial if the child could join a drama club at school or one of the theatre schools such as *Stagecoach*, which devotes an hour to dancing, an hour to singing and an hour to drama in each three-hour class, and accepts everyone without audition (details in *Further Resources*). (My daughter joined and loves it; she is brave enough to go on her own and has also coped with changing schools when a class closer to home started. She has made her own friends there, none of whom go to her school.)

CHANGING NEGATIVE THOUGHTS

Negative thoughts are extremely unhelpful and are the root of many ills. Once the negative thought is identified, alternative helpful thoughts can be created. For example, a social phobic child may have negative thoughts about going to a party. She should write down these negative thoughts and think of alternative, positive thoughts she could use:

1. If I go, there will be no one to talk to.

   Alternative thought: If I don't go, there'll be no one to talk to. I may meet someone interesting that I have something in common with.

2. I've not got anything interesting to say. No one will talk to me for long.

   Alternative thought: It doesn't matter that I don't have anything interesting to say – other people often have and I'm a good listener. People do like to talk about themselves.

3. I can never remember other people's names when they are introduced to me.

   Alternative thought: They probably can't remember mine either. If I get to talk to someone that I've previously been introduced to, I can ask for his name again. It makes it easier to remember if I repeat it, especially if I'm not sure of the pronunciation. If it's a name I've not come across before I could ask how it's spelt. For most if not all people, their name is the most important word in their life. They'll be happy that I'm making an effort to get it right.

4. I won't be able to think of anything to say.

    Alternative thought: I can prepare questions to ask that I could ask anyone and use these each time I meet someone new. The questions can be about family and pets, hobbies, holidays, favourite and least favourite subjects, and whether the person has a part-time job. I can also have ready some basic information about myself that I don't mind sharing.

5. I'll make a fool of myself so there's no point in going.

    Alternative thought: I'll make a fool of myself by not going as people will know that I've made yet another excuse. Everyone makes mistakes and I can laugh mine off.

6. I don't feel well (with general anxiety-related malaise), so I'm sure I'll feel far worse if I go.

    Alternative thought: I don't feel well because I've worked myself up into a state of anxiety. As soon as I relax I will feel better. And the sooner I get there, the sooner that will happen. The thought is more frightening than the event because of magnifying my own problems and inadequacies in my mind.

7. I've only been invited to make up numbers. The host doesn't really want to see me.

    Alternative thought: If the host really doesn't want me there, it won't make much difference if I spill something. It takes away some of the pressure as his attention won't be focused on me. And so what if I was invited to make up numbers? It doesn't mean I can't go and enjoy myself.

8. I usually come away from these things feeling bad about myself. It would be better if I stayed at home.

    Alternative thought: If I put more effort into getting involved with other people I'll have a nicer time and feel better about myself. It's only because I wouldn't talk to anyone that didn't talk to me first that I felt bad afterwards.

9. Someone might tease me if I make a mess of things such as spill my food or drink on myself.

    Alternative thought: It is usually a compliment if I'm teased because it means that someone feels comfortable enough in my presence to feel able to do it. Otherwise they wouldn't bother. No one is likely to be unkind to me when they don't know me. And it might mean the person fancies me because teasing can be a form of flirting (together with other body language hints).

10. I'm worried that my hand will shake when I pick up my glass and that others will notice.

    Alternative thought: Why should I feel that everyone is watching what I do? There are so many people at parties that their attention, if on others, will be spread around. I can always limit the number of times I pick up my drink. And if I find someone else to talk to, I'll be too interested in the conversation to worry about my hands.

11. I hate parties because I'm a useless dancer.

    Alternative thought: If I practise at home in front of dance videos or *Top of the Pops*, or with friends, I'll get better. I might never be great, but dancing is about having fun and enjoying myself. (There are now dancing machines available in amusement arcades that can help children practise pop routines.)

Other helpful thoughts about going to a party:

- It's dark at parties so if I blush, no one will know.

- There are buffets at parties so if I feel too anxious to eat, I don't have to. I could always eat before I leave home.

- If I find it hard to talk to someone I can suggest we dance. (Social phobia is different for each sufferer. There are some things that one social phobic can do that another finds impossible and vice versa. Each group of worries differs for each person. So some are happier to dance than talk. For others, they prefer talking to dancing.)

The child should learn helpful statements so that she can say them like a mantra when necessary. And if she says them at other times too, it will help her believe them. She has much work to do to undo all the damage her negative thoughts have done, as repeating them many times has made her believe them.

The child should be warned about the times when she might be particularly vulnerable to negative thoughts, so that she can be prepared for setbacks and make an extra effort to banish the negative thoughts from her mind. Such times might be: when she is ill or is recovering from illness, when something has gone wrong, when she's been disappointed about something or when she feels overwhelmed by her life. At these times, no major decisions should be made at all. She should wait until she feels fully recovered and then look at the dilemma objectively, writing down all the pros and cons.

Conclusion

Social anxieties are very common. It has been estimated[12] that up to 40 per cent of people have some form of social anxiety. In Japan, it has been reported that one million young men[13] suffer a form of social withdrawal called *hikikomori*, where they shut themselves away in a room (usually a bedroom) for years; their families hide the problem so as not to risk social embarrassment. This is an extreme form of social phobia peculiar to Japan.

The fears socially anxious people have are never allayed by avoidance of situations; doing so only allows the fears to grow and take firm hold. They are best dealt with by as much exposure to social situations as possible, including those that cause the greatest anxiety. However, gradual desensitisation is usually the best approach, with the understanding and support of those around the child who experiences the difficulties.

References

1.   mentalhelp.net/disorders/sx35.htm

2.   www.familymedicine.co.uk/novarticles/socphobia.htm

3.   www.mcmaster.ca/inabis98/ameringen/oakman0804/two.html

4. www.selectivemutismfoundation.org/frameset.html

5. www.members.tripod.com/ernallo/possible1.htm

6. www.selectivemutism.org/main12.htm

7. www.members.tripod.com/ernallo/presenta.htm

8. www.findarticles.com/cf_0/m0[HVD]/2_22/75562745/p5/article. j html?term=

9. www.members.tripod.com/ernallo

10. www.findarticles.com/cf_0/m0[HVD]/2_22/75562745/p4/article. j html?term=

11. www.nas.org.uk/pubs/faqs/qsleep.html

12. www.anxietycare.org.uk

13. *Correspondent* BBC 2 (20 October 2002), reported in *Radio Times*, 19–25 October 2002.

Further reading

Web addresses for further information and advice on selective mutism:

www.adaa.org/anxietydisorderinfor/childrenado.cfm#sm (Anxiety Disorders Association of America's website on anxiety disorders, including selective mutism.)

www.selectivemutism.org

www.selective-mutism.com

www.asha.org/speech/disabilities/selective-mutism.cfm (American Speech-Language-Hearing Association website.)

www.aboutourkids.org/articles/about_mutism.html (New York University Child Study Center website.)

Web addresses for further information and advice on social phobia:

www.socialphobia.org/fact.html#top (Social Phobia/Social Anxiety Association website, based in the US.)

www.ability.org.uk/social_phobia.html (Ability website: 'see the ability not the disability'.)

www.phobics-society.org.uk (National Phobics Society website.)

www.adaa.org/anxietydisorderinfor/childrenado.cfm (Anxiety
Disorders Association of America's webpages on anxiety disorders and
social anxiety in children and adolescents.)

www.une.edu.au/psychology/staff/malouff/shyness.htm#what
(Details the methods used to socialise a very shy child. Written by a
lecturer in psychology.)

Web addresses for more information on *hikikomori*:

www.csmonitor.com/durable/2000/08/16/p1s4.htm

www.time.com/time/asia/magazine/2000/0501/
japan.essaymurakami.html

Books

Csóti, M. (1997) *Assertiveness Skills For Young Adults.* Corby, UK: First & Best
    in Education.
This is a simple assertiveness training course designed to be used in school
sixth forms, but can be used by parents and other professionals with young
people aged 15 plus. (The student sheets are photocopiable for group work.)
No expertise is needed as full guidance is given in the book.

Berent, J. and Lemley, A. (1994) *Beyond Shyness: How to Conquer Social
    Anxieties.* New York: Simon & Schuster.
This book includes sections on helping children and teenagers with social
anxiety and avoidance, with special advice for parents.

Butler, G. (1999) *Overcoming Social Anxiety and Shyness.* London: Robinson.
This is a self-help manual for adults, but is useful in understanding social
unease and, through the reader, can help younger children.

Csóti, M. (1999) *People Skills for Young Adults.* London: Jessica Kingsley
    Publishers.
This is a social skills training course for young people aged 16 and above and is
particularly suited to those with mild learning difficulties. If the child has poor
social skills or would like to improve the quality of her social interactions, this
book offers interesting role-plays and discussions. No expertise is needed to
run the sessions as full guidance is given in the book.

Csóti, M. (2001) *Social Awareness Skills for Children.* London: Jessica Kingsley Publishers.
This is a very comprehensive social skills course for parents and professionals to follow with children aged 7 to 16, using many role-plays and discussions. It can be used with children who have specific difficulties in picking up social skills because of a medical problem (such as Asperger syndrome), but the book is also an invaluable resource to use with any child, particularly for unconfident children who are social phobic. No expertise is needed as full guidance is given in the book.

Csóti, M. (2003) *The People Skills Bible.* Cardiff: Welsh Academic Press.
This is a self-improvement book that gives very comprehensive guidance on all aspects of social interaction for the older adolescent and adults generally. It will help readers gain social confidence to overcome shyness and social anxiety and heighten their social awareness so that, in time, they can become advanced players. It has something in it for everyone, thus professionals can use it with their clients, and parents with their children, by passing on information and tips.

Csóti, M. (2001) *Contentious Issues: Discussion Stories for Young People.* London: Jessica Kingsley Publishers.
This book has 40 stories tackling personal social and health education issues, with discussion questions and full leader support. It is designed to help children become socially responsible, empathetic adults while learning about life skills and life choices and the consequences of their actions and inactions. Discussing issues in a friendly environment will help children to talk more freely about the same issues in a less secure environment and will enable them to explore issues, so that they develop their own opinions and will feel comfortable voicing them to other people. It will help social phobic children and those who have poor communication skills.

Chapter Six

Positively Dealing with the Child's Anxieties

Anxiety can interfere hugely with the child's life and is hard to deal with because parents do not always know why she is anxious. It is very distressing for parents and the child when she is unhappy about going to school, but even more so when this reluctance becomes so great it affects her health and social interactions.

Below are suggestions to help the child; they should be adapted to suit her particular problems and circumstances, and her age. Some suggestions are only applicable to the very young and some suggestions are only for parents to think about.

Don't be part of the problem
Unwittingly, parents may have contributed to the child's reliance on them; there are many ways in which this can happen.

When a child is ill or has a medical condition
Parents may be over-anxious for the child and attempt to over-compensate for her troubles, feeling guilty that she is not experiencing the same sort of life as her friends. For example, if a child has a particular health problem or has been admitted to hospital, parents may feel so grateful that she has come through that they lavish her with affection and attention. This can then continue after she is over the ordeal. The same can happen if a child has suffered a long illness through which

164

parents have nursed her. It may be hard to withdraw this extra attention when the child becomes well again, prolonging her need for her parents.

If a child becomes so emotionally dependent on her parents that she must have them close by even when she is well, she has regressed from the stage of development she was at before her illness. This makes it harder for her to return to school and accept the school environment once more, remembering how warm and secure she felt at home with her parents close by and checking on her, giving her treats. Children, like adults who have become institutionalised, can lose their independence and their self-confidence. This immediately compounds the problems of separation anxiety and school phobia.

New fears should not be introduced because of parental worries

Parents should try to remove any unnecessary pressure from the child as she needs to be protected from stress regardless of how they feel. For example, if parents are concerned about the child's weight and they weigh her, it should have no more significance to her than their brushing her teeth. Her weight is unlikely to change much daily; weighing her more than once a week is not likely to give parents any extra information and is likely to make the child anxious. If she wants to know how much she weighs, parents could tell her. But they should not frighten her by telling her that she is losing weight and she'll be ill if she can't eat.

Parents can do all the worrying for the child. If she is underweight but stable, there is not a great deal to worry about. As long as the child is drinking plenty, she will stay fairly healthy. If parents are very worried about her weight, or are concerned she may be developing an eating disorder, they should consult the child's doctor.

Neither should parents discourage the child from doing things she wants to because they worry how she'll cope, knowing she's an anxious child. This will only increase her anxiety and make her more dependent on them.

Neither the child nor the parents should be blamed for her problems

The problem needs to be understood without casting blame. If the child's parents don't understand it, they should just do their best to accept the child's difficulties and help her through them. Very often, the cause is only understood when parents look back, after it is all over. They might be so entrenched in worrying that they are unable to stand back and look at the problem objectively. With some children, the cause might never be known.

Parents should not be overheard talking to others

Parents should not speak to others about the child's problems within earshot of the child unless it is in the most casual of ways. She should not pick up on their anxiety through an in-depth conversation, nor should she be subjected to other people's surprise or shock. She needs to be protected from these reactions, otherwise she might see her problems as even bigger than before. She needs to feel secure, knowing that her parents are in control. They can admit to not having all the answers, needing outside help and trying things out to see what might help her, as long as she does not realise how scared and worried they might be. It was mentioned earlier that the way the parent reacts to the child witnessing or experiencing a traumatic event has enormous influence on how the child herself is affected. If they don't feel confident and in control of the situation, they should try to hide it.

Parents should not ignore unacceptable behaviour

The child needs to know that the ground rules remain the same. Parents can become softer in their approach, but the child's anxieties should not become an excuse for her to become spoilt and to do as she pleases whenever she pleases. This would make it a bigger shock to her when things get back to 'normal' and she has another adjustment to make.

Parents should try to be gentle, but remain firm about things they know they would never allow the child to do if she weren't having problems. It is more reassuring to the child to have the same boundaries as before she became anxious, and she may deliberately test these to check that they haven't changed. Children find comfort and security in familiarity and rules they know and understand.

Parents should not be critical of the child's school or her teachers

Another thing parents need to watch out for is criticising the child's school or teachers in front of her. They need to speak only positively about the place in her hearing or she will think it's not a good place to be. If they have a problem with something the teacher does, they should go directly to the teacher to discuss it. This is especially important in primary school, where a child spends most of the week with her class teacher. In secondary school, a child has so many teachers that slight parental criticism of one may be balanced by positive comments about the rest.

Positive things to do to help an anxious child

The anxious child will be feeling lost and bewildered and desperately needs to feel comforted and understood. Below are some suggestions to help make this a less traumatic time for the child.

Reassure the child

The child should be reassured that her anxious feelings won't be with her all the time; she'll feel better once she's got over the part she dreads.

Explain things

The child should have it explained that everyone feels anxious about things at times; life isn't always easy. And if she fears being sick, she can be told that no one likes being sick: it's a horrible thing to experience, but it's a part of how people's bodies behave when ill or worried and it only lasts a short time. The only way to stop things worrying her is for her to get on and do things in spite of how she feels or what happens. It's her own private battle and she needs to be brave and overcome her fear. (Also see *Cognitive therapy* in Chapter Seven.)

Show the child life goes on regardless

When the child is in great distress, adults should not make a drama out of it. The child should be talked to in a down-to-earth way so that she is soothed by how calm her carers are. Her fears should not prevent others from doing things in the way they normally would. Not carrying on regardless makes the child think that she's got an insurmountable problem to which the whole family must adapt to fulfil her needs. This only makes her more insecure.

Tell the child how brave she is

It is easy for the child's friends to go to school, but for her it's the hardest thing she's come across. She should be told how proud her parents are of her for being so brave.

Tell the child she is loved

The child will be feeling very insecure and she needs to know that she is not in trouble for her behaviour and that she is not being punished for it. She needs to understand that her parents' love for her is unconditional: that whatever she does, they will still love her.

Give the child plenty of physical affection

The child needs to have words of love from her parents reinforced by physical affection. This gives her comfort and security at a time when she needs it most. She may become clingy and want to be cuddled all the time. As long as parents can give her a good measure of affection every day, at different times in the day, the child will feel loved. She may need to be near them, following them from room to room; they should try to accept this.

When parents cook, for example, the child could draw or paint in the kitchen (or in the doorway if there isn't room) so that she is near them and does not feel rejected. Allowances should be made for her insecurity and craving for comfort. She must not be rejected.

Make bedtime special

Bedtime can be an anxious time and the child may find it hard to sleep because of worry. She may have experienced great relief in coming home, but going to bed marks the end of the day and the 'relaxed time' she had when she first came home from school, and reminds her that after sleep comes the next hurdle.

BEDTIME STORIES

Parents should cuddle the child in bed and read her a bedtime story if she is very young. They should spend time listening to her and talking to her. This is a special time for them to share with her. They should try to reassure the child about how she is doing.

If the child is over 10 and bedtime stories are a thing of the past, parents could have special books for her to read that are only for bedtime. If she is put to bed before she needs to settle down, she can have a quiet time enjoying the story. Keeping her mind occupied on a good story (but one that is not too gripping as she doesn't need to be more stimulated) may distract her from her worries.

Cassette recordings and dramatisations of books can be borrowed from the local library as an alternative to reading, or to add variety to the bedtime routine. The advantage of these is that they can be listened to after the light has been switched off.

Being caught up in an interesting world might give wonderful relief to the child's overtaxed mind, and the more absorbed she is in the stories, the better. If reserved as a bedtime treat, she may not dread the time so much.

PLAY HER RELAXING CASSETTES/CDS

Parents could play cassettes/CDs of soft relaxing music for a young child to fall asleep to. These again help to distract her mind so that it can switch off, relax and let go of the day's upsets. And, for older children who can be taught relaxation techniques, parents could buy or borrow special relaxation cassettes/CDs that teach them how to breathe diaphragmatically and how to systematically tense and relax their muscles so that they can achieve deep relaxation. (See *Further Resources.*)

When using relaxation/sleep cassettes/CDs, it is a good idea to have either a cassette or CD player close to hand for the child to listen to, or headphones connected to a portable player in bed with the (older) child. The child does not have to have sleep problems to benefit from relaxation cassettes/CDs.

Before a relaxation/sleep cassette/CD is given to the child, parents should listen to and work through it themselves or do it with the child. It is vital that they know and understand what deep relaxation feels like. If they work through the cassette/CD at bedtime, they will also notice how much more refreshed they are in the morning. How this feels should be explained to the child so that she knows what she is working towards; it does require effort to follow cassettes/CDs and to concentrate on what she's asked to do. When followed regularly, they can change her (and her parents') life.

LISTEN TO WHAT THE CHILD WANTS

If parents can make things easier for the child, they should do so. For example, she may suddenly want to have a light on when she's been going to sleep for years in the dark. Or she might need to have them close by and her anxiety about them not being within calling distance may make her too worried to fall asleep. Parents should comply with the child's wishes as far as they possibly can, as going to bed is a lonely thing for a child who feels vulnerable and scared.

If the child is sensitive to light and noise (children with autistic spectrum disorders can have sensitivities to these, and to touch), it would help to black out her bedroom so that the light does not prevent her from sleeping, and for the rest of the house to become quiet once the child is in bed (and during the winding-down period before bed). If the child is sensitive to touch, parents should investigate what arrangement of bedclothes and nightwear suits her best: how many layers and what material she can tolerate.

Food sensitivities may also interfere with the child's ability to sleep. Drinks containing caffeine are best not taken at bedtime (and could be changed to a non-caffeine brand). Better still, children should avoid any food or drink that acts as a stimulant as this can increase their anxiety during the day.

Have a gentle start to the day

It should be understood that the child may not want to get up in the mornings, out of the warmth and security of her bed, fearing the day ahead. A gentle start to the day – being woken by relaxing music, a much-loved pet or cuddles – may help the child accept that it is morning and that the routine of the day must begin.

Get the child up early

The child should have plenty of time before school so that the prepara-tions run smoothly and without rushing. She needs to be told that she has to be dressed by a certain time (if she has motor skills problems, getting dressed may take her a long time), to have finished her breakfast by a certain time, etc. and this should be kept to every day. The child may feel anxious at the thought of being late, so a calm and measured pace each morning is essential.

Keep to the same routine

The child should have, as far as possible, the same basic routine in holiday time as she does in term time: getting up and going to bed at the same times as she would if she were going to school. This gives her less change when school starts again, so she doesn't have to suddenly adjust to a new routine and cope with being tired because she was unable to sleep at the right time.

Children with autistic spectrum disorders rely heavily on rigid routines to cope with their anxiety (see chapters One and Two). Any deviation from what the child expects can lead to panic, so routine is even more vital to such a child.

ROUTINE TO HELP SLEEP

The child should also have a set bedtime routine: the order of tea, washing, quiet time (for winding down), bedtime story, etc. This is a time of insecurity in the child's life and she needs to feel enclosed in a safe and comforting place. Routine is boring but will increase her feeling of security because of its familiarity.

Some children with autistic spectrum disorders are anxious about going to sleep and often don't get enough sleep (although a few sleep too much), perceiving sleep as a dark nothingness that steals over them, outside of their control. They may have very disturbing nightmares, which can make them anxious for future bedtimes. They may also not see the point of going to sleep at a particular time, not understanding that it is the norm for people to sleep at night and for the child to be asleep before, or at the same time as, his parents. It should be explained that this is a routine the family sticks to because it is sensible to sleep at the end of the day, to have energy for the next and for everyone to sleep at the same time to keep the house quiet: adults need less sleep than children, thus go to bed later so that everyone can wake up at the same time (assuming no one does shift work).[1]

Reduce the number of things the child needs to worry about

The child will already have an over-active mind if she is in a constant state of anxiety. Parents should do whatever they can to prevent other worries being added. For example, they should let her see that every-thing is ready for the morning – her clothes, sandwiches/lunch money, homework. If her hair might need washing, it shouldn't be done in a rush just before school, but washed the night before.

If there is anything particularly upsetting happening in the news (murders, major rail or 'plane crashes, school coach crashes, missing children, natural disasters), the child shouldn't hear about it or see it on television, or in a newspaper. Nor should the child watch frightening films or programmes; details from these can stick in her mind, which is vulnerable to negative thoughts and susceptible to worry.

AVOID UNCERTAINTIES WHENEVER POSSIBLE

If the child has an appointment, exactly what is going to happen should be explained. For example, who will pick her up, when, and at what time she'll be back in school. If parents are unsure whether she will make it for lunch, instead of saying to her, 'You'll have lunch in school if we're back in time, otherwise we'll take you home,' they should tell her that they'll definitely have lunch at home and return her to school at the end of lunch break. The uncertainty of not knowing whether she'll be back in school may make her watch the clock anxiously, wondering whether she'll make it and worrying that the teacher might be annoyed with her for missing lunch as she'd booked it. Parents should avoid uncertainties whenever possible.

Enlist the help of the other members of the family

Each member of the family could be told exactly what they can do to help; examples are:

- Avoid mentioning school to the child, unless she brings up the subject first.

- Ignore the number of times the child goes to the toilet.

- Avoid talking about being sick, vomit and diarrhoea.

- Avoid all teasing; the child feels bad enough already.

- Try to be kind and say nice things to the child; it will help raise her self-esteem at a time when her confidence is low. She needs to feel valued by all.

- Try to distract the child by reading her (happy) stories or by playing involving or fun games with her. The less time the child spends thinking about school, the more chance she has to let her body unwind and reach a semblance of calm.

- Try to keep the family atmosphere as normal as possible. For example, if the family suddenly stop talking the moment the child walks into the room, she will know they have all been talking about her.

- Try to minimise the child's thoughts of school and her problems. If she thinks family members don't find it too big a problem, she might worry less herself (but they shouldn't pretend her problems don't exist).

Protect the child from extended family members and friends

The child's problems should also be explained to extended family members and friends and they should be asked not to talk about school to the child unless she brings up the topic first. The child might be thinking about it so often, she might not find further reminders helpful.

They should also be asked to ignore any strange behaviour that is part of the child's anxiety (such as multiple visits to the toilet). They should not tease her about it or make her feel bad about it in any way.

They should not say unhelpful things such as, 'Don't you think it's time you stopped this nonsense?' or 'Pull yourself together, girl. We didn't behave like this in my day' or 'You think you've got problems? You don't know what problems are. You've not had a real problem in your life.' Other people need to accept the child as she is and not make any judgements.

Help from extended family members and friends

It would help the child if parents could increase the number of adults the child trusts enough to be taken out with. This will push back some of her boundaries and make her more confident at coping without the presence of her parents.

Talk to her friends

The child's problems could be explained to some of her closer friends and they could be told how to help: by looking after her when she gets to school and by being kind to her. It is very hard for young children to empathise, so this might need to be spelt out.

For teenagers, it is best not to talk to friends unless given permission to by the child. It may make the problem worse if the child feels more self-conscious because more people know. If the problem is obvious to everyone, however, the child should give parents permission to suggest ways her friends could help, because that is what they are supposed to do (and the child would want to help her friends if they had problems).

Reassess the rules parents expect the child to observe

Parents should question things that are rules for the sake of them. Being firm does not mean parents can't change their mind about rules the child has now outgrown, or rules that are inherited from their own parents and are no longer relevant. They should watch the number of times they criticise the child when she breaks rules, and consider if it is worth having an unimportant rule that makes the child feel bad about herself whenever she breaks it.

Treat the child each school day

Parents should allow the child to have or do something pleasurable each school day to give her something to look forward to and enjoy. This is particularly important if she shows signs of depression. The child needs to keep experiencing love and care through what her parents do for her.

She mustn't lose touch with the external world and withdraw into her own miserable world where she cannot be reached.

Give her reasons to look forward to going to school

Parents could buy special clothes just for school or, if the child has a school uniform, buy something special that's just for use in school, such as a new pencil case with pens and pencils. If she has a new school bag that she helped choose she may enjoy packing her things in it. Parents could sometimes hide a small gift in her bag so that she comes across it during the day, such as a new rubber or a wrapped chocolate biscuit.

Make up charts for the child

Parents could use a chart (there is a template to photocopy at the end of this chapter) to record the child's feelings each morning (including the weekends). There are no right and wrong answers but she can still be rewarded by having a sticker put on the days she has positive feelings, such as feeling relaxed, happy, excited, eager, etc. This will help her to feel important by parents caring enough to ask her how she felt during the day, and it takes the pressure off being a success or a failure. For example, if she were rewarded for each day she didn't have a panic attack, managed to eat her breakfast or didn't throw up, she would feel pressurised into succeeding at these things and that pressure would make it less likely for her to achieve the unachievable. It is how the child feels that holds the key. Once her feelings become more positive, the rest will follow.

Parents could use another chart (there is a template to photocopy at the end of this chapter) as a display to remind the child about the week. They could have a column for each day of the week and ask the child to think of something she likes to do on that particular day, then record it after the name of the day. The more positive things the child can think of the better. An example might be:

Monday: Painting.

Tuesday: Singing.

Wednesday: Having friend to tea.

Thursday: Watch children's programme in school.

Friday: Fish and chips for school dinner.

Saturday: Go shopping for food. I get an ice cream.

Sunday: Having a special lunch. Visiting Grandma.

Things that are the same most days should be avoided, for example, watching television at home: this is a very passive activity, requiring no effort on the child's part. The positive things should be active and, preferably on school days, she should think of at least one thing she likes in school time. However, this may not be immediate. If she can't think of anything for one of the days, the child could be challenged to think of something she quite likes doing during that school day. It may be sitting at lunch with friends, or story time. No matter how small the thing is, it is the first building brick of a change in attitude.

For older children they might enjoy after-school clubs, individual subjects or the journey home when they mess about with their friends. Or there might be a particular friend they enjoy seeing, and being in school allows that to happen more frequently.

If the child's week changes from week to week, parents could have a separate chart for each week. When each day comes, the child should be reminded about the things she has to look forward to, whether something in school or after school. These may help her focus her mind when at school and gradually shift her thoughts from all negative to some positive. As she starts to feel more positive about her days, and hopefully her time in school, she may become aware of other things that she enjoys and can then add these to the list, creating a circle of positive feedback so that her thoughts become more and more positive.

Parents should show the child that they look forward to things. They could mention some things they don't like very much, adding that these make them appreciate the good things even more and that they think of these good things when they have to do things they don't like. This is part of life. (But parents shouldn't make adult life sound depressing; they should note the positive points of living independently too.)

Help the child to play using her fears

Parents may be able to help a young child through the medium of play. The child's favourite cuddly toy can have 'tummy ache' just like the child and can be afraid to go to school. If parents show how to reassure the anxious toy, the child may copy them and in doing so use helpful thoughts that become more imprinted in her own mind. Cuddling a toy at night that has the same problems as the child might be very comforting to her.

And if the child has a bad day but won't tell her parents why, they could ask her if her toy has had a bad day too. She may tell her parents what has upset the toy, giving them the information they need to help her. They can then ask the child how she thinks the toy can be helped. In this way, she may work out what she has to do herself.

Praise the child for small achievements

No matter how small the progress, if the child has succeeded in doing something without mishap or succeeded in doing it without as much agony as before, she should be praised. She needs these positive comments for the times when she finds things hard. Knowing that parents are proud of her for her efforts gives her courage to continue.

Try to keep out-of-school hours as normal as possible

If the child used to have friends round to play, parents should keep inviting them. If she used to go to other people's homes but now doesn't want to, it could be explained to their parents why she can't and their children could be invited to the child's place instead. It is important that she maintains some social contact so that she doesn't become socially isolated. It also helps reduce depression. Bonding in a non-stressful environment will help her cope better when she sees the friends at school and they will be more interested in supporting her.

Keep an eye on the child's health

Remember the boy who cried 'wolf'? No one believed him because he had done it too many times when nothing was wrong. Parents should try not to let that happen to the child. One day, she really will be ill when she says she feels ill. It is good to have a checklist of things to monitor, such as:

- Does the child have a temperature? A quick check can be done by parents kissing the back of the child's neck or touching it with their hand. Feeling very warm skin does not probably suggest a temperature but when parents start to feel that the skin is hot, there might be. A high temperature is obvious because the skin will feel extremely hot. Then parents can check with a thermometer.

- Has the child got a sore throat? This can be checked using a teaspoon to depress the child's tongue and a torch to illuminate the back of her throat. (A sore throat shows up as a darker pink than the surrounding flesh. If the throat is very sore it may look red.) If the child has white spots on her tonsils, she's probably got tonsillitis and will need to see a doctor. Viral pharyngitis can give white spots on the child's palate.

- If the child has stomachache, is it a general ache or is it a sharp pain that has persisted for some hours? Is the pain in one place or does it move around? Is the child vague about where it hurts? Sharp persistent pain will need to be checked by her doctor.

- A young child should be asked seriously if her left knee hurts too. If she's making up the stomach pain, she might say she's got pain elsewhere and hopefully will be unaware that they are unconnected and that parents are testing her. If parents do this, they should never tell her that it's not serious because she can't possibly have a pain in her left knee as well as her stomach, etc. She should just be told that it's nothing to worry about. The pain will go away.

- Is the child constipated? Parents can sometimes feel this if the child lies relaxed on the bed with her hands by her sides. If they gently depress her abdomen with flattened fingers rather than points, they should be able to feel sausage shaped lumps, or the belly might be bloated all over. If it is soft and yielding there is less chance the child is constipated. Please note that no one should ever press hard or press on an area over which there is sharp pain, as it could injure the child. For example, it might burst her appendix or another organ where there is infection or obstruction.

- If the child has a headache, is she dehydrated? (If in doubt, she could be given a large drink of water.) Has the child bumped her head? Has she other symptoms such as a sore throat and runny nose or a high temperature? Blocked sinuses can cause headaches and these are generally nothing to worry about. (Occasionally the sinuses become infected and need to be treated.)

- Is anything happening (different to other times) that could be causing her symptoms? Is something new coming along, or does the child have no cause for extra anxiety? If not, her symptoms might indicate the early stages of illness.

Adults should never give medical information that's unnecessary to a child. For example, if the child knows about appendicitis and thinks because she has a pain she has it, adults shouldn't tell her that it can't be because this is where appendicitis pain would be. The next time she might develop pain there just because she's anxious about it and then parents won't know whether it's a genuine cause for concern.

RELIEVING THE CHILD'S ANXIETIES ABOUT BEING IN PAIN

If the child is anxious about abdominal pain (or any other pain) it should initially be checked out. If parents are not worried they should tell the child that if the pain gets worse or moves, to let them know and then they'll have another look. (Sometimes appendicitis can start in the middle and then move sharply down.) If parents are not sure about stomach pains, they should ask the child's doctor to explain what needs to be looked at and what doesn't. Usually, these pains are nothing to worry about and reassurance is all that the child needs, plus a possible explanation, such as she's probably hungry or constipated, or her glands are swollen because she has a virus, or she's picked up a virus that gives her stomachache. She should be told that sometimes people get stomachache and there is no apparent reason for it.

A genuinely unwell child should not be forced to push herself beyond comfortable limits, even though adults may choose to do this. If a child has severe pain that has previously been checked out (such as colic-type pain when she has a virus from swollen glands in the abdomen), parents should let her rest. Parents can check that the pain is attributable to swollen glands by checking her throat. If it is red then she probably does have a virus. If it is its normal light pink colour then there may be another cause, which could be anxiety.

Every time the anxious child comes up with a fresh pain, parents need to show her that they've listened to what she has to say and then tell her it's nothing to worry about. They could say, 'Thank you for telling me. There's nothing to worry about now. If it changes, let me know.' Then the child has given parents the responsibility of worrying about the pain and can go away relieved that she is not about to collapse from some serious illness. If parents ignore her fears completely, she may worry all the more that there is something wrong, be upset because she feels her parents didn't listen, and keep worrying about it until it is dealt with.

Parents should be aware of the possibility of period pain once the girl has started her periods. Some girls get sharp pain in the middle of the month when they ovulate (and this can be confused with appendicitis if the pain is in the right ovary). Usually, the severity of the pain is short-lived if it's from ovulation and may settle after half an hour. Continuous severe pain should never be ignored and parents should consult the child's doctor.

Spend some time alone each day with the child

Parents should have a special, quiet time when they cuddle up with the child and talk about the child's day. This may be hard if parents have other children and lead a hectic life – but it is important. Likewise, parents mustn't forget other children if they have them, or they will feel resentful towards the child who has the problems.

Confide problems to people parents trust

Confiding allows parents to get emotional support and possibly useful suggestions or an introduction to a recommended professional. Parents can support the child more effectively if they are not working alone. This is a stressful time for parents as well as for the child, and they too need support.

Speak to the child's teacher and headteacher

The child's teacher and headteacher should be asked if they can help in some way. Do they have suggestions? Have they come across similar problems before? Could the child eat her breakfast when she arrives in school or at first break (if she vomits every morning or is too nauseous to eat)? Other suggestions, for very young children are:

- Could someone meet the child as she comes off the bus?

- Could she be sat with a friend on the way home?

- Could someone look after the child when she arrives in school, and comfort her when she is sick and help her clean up? Then give her a drink? Although children shouldn't be made to be more dependent on adults, young children need help and reassurance. Coping on her own may give the child confidence because she did manage it, but it may make her feel that no one in the school cares about her.

- Could she be reassured and cuddled when she arrives?

- Could the school secretary ring up once the class teacher feels that the child is relaxed and interacting normally, to stop parents worrying about her all day?

- Could parents have a report of what she eats at lunchtime (without the child's knowledge)?

- Could teachers tell the child's parents what she does at break times? Does she run around and play games? Is she alone? Does she try to stay in the cloakroom?

School staff don't always appreciate the devastating effect school phobia can have on the whole family. It is better to share the responsibility of the child's unhappiness and have home and school both work together to solve it.

Monitor the child's progress

The child can become anxious if there is work at school that she cannot do. If parents ask the child about her day and listen to what she says, this can be picked up on early. Checking that the child is comfortable with the work she is given is very important. If she feels unable to cope with her work, she will not enjoy school.

If the child is behind her peers in her work, her teacher could be asked to lend parents the materials they need (such as a maths workbook) and to let parents know how they can help. Being helped at home helps the child to feel comfortable about the academic side of school, as she is not likely to worry about sitting in front of a page of seemingly nonsensical writing and numbers.

However, helping the child should not be taken to an extreme. It is not good for the child if parents push her academically, and if she goes too far ahead of her class she might find the work she does in school boring. But there is no harm in her reading slightly ahead of what the class will be doing, to introduce the child to new topics. The advantage of this is that when the child comes across that particular area again in school, it helps consolidate what she has begun and she might reach a more thorough understanding. She may then also feel very proud of herself for managing to do something in class on her own.

Conclusion

Hopefully, after some time, the child will relax enough to get fed up with playing on her own, knowing her friends are partying and having fun. It may take months and improvement may be very gradual, but eventually the child should tire of having a very boring life (although at the beginning this is what she craves and needs to make her feel more secure). However, the child can only be pushed forward if she is receiving genuine help from all sides, otherwise there is a risk of making the situation worse, increasing her stress.

The pace at which parents work is dependent on family circumstances, the child's personality and degree of anxiety, and the opportunities that come their way. For example, if the child gets invited to one party a year, there is not much opportunity to get her desensitised to going to parties and being left there. If there are three or more a term, it's worth using them to enlarge the boundaries of the child's independence. Adults should proceed gently and not expect things to magically change. They should accept that extreme anxiety can take a long time to beat.

Reference

1.   www.nas.org.uk/pubs/faqs/qsleep.html

My Feelings Chart

	Monday	Tuesday	Wednesday	Thursday	Friday	Saturday	Sunday
Week 1							
Week 2							
Week 3							
Week 4							
Week 5							
Week 6							
Week 7							

My Chart to Show the Things I Enjoy	
	The things I enjoy or look forward to
Mondays	
Tuesdays	
Wednesdays	
Thursdays	
Fridays	
Saturdays	
Sundays	

Chapter Seven

When the Child is Severely Affected by Anxiety and Related Problems

A child is severely affected by anxiety and related problems when her worries and symptoms affect her everyday life and, if she is not improving or her symptoms have lasted more than a few weeks, the most appropriate action is for her to be referred to a professional. Referrals can take a while if there is a long waiting list; during the wait the child's problems may escalate (although they can resolve), so it is better for the child to be referred before she becomes so unwell that she cannot attend school at all. Child and adolescent mental health professionals often prioritise school refusal of short duration to 'nip it in the bud' before it becomes a long-standing problem.

Professional help is important because parents need to know they are doing the right things; they might be given advice on things they have not yet thought of and they need to know what to avoid so as not to make things worse or prolong the child's problems.

Parents also need support. They need to know that they are not the only parents who have gone through this and that their child isn't so odd that no other child has experienced similar difficulties. They also need to know that they are not to blame. (Blame is not seen as a useful tool by child and adolescent mental health professionals.) Parents also need to be reassured about the situation and need to be encouraged to take steps they may be frightened of taking; that is, being cruel to be kind.

Many parents balk at the idea of asking for a referral to a mental health specialist, because of the stigma that continues to be attached to people in need of such help, yet this may be just what the child needs. Anxiety disorders can be debilitating for children and adolescents, and stressful for families. Prompt, appropriate treatment can be effective in alleviating the symptoms and helping the child return to normal functioning without long-term harm.

Seeking professional help

The first step in seeking outside help is for parents to talk to the child's teachers, since many of the child's difficulties may centre around going to and attending school. They should discuss the child's problems with relatives, friends and neighbours who might have known other children in similar situations. If they have a religious leader whom they are close to, parents may feel that he or she can offer help or advice.

If these avenues have not provided a solution for the child, the next step is to seek trained professional help. The child's general practitioner can give an initial assessment and reassure parents that there is no physical problem. This is also important if the child is missing school. A diagnosis from a doctor proves that the child is not truanting and that the absences are authorised. It also confirms that the child needs specialist help. If the doctor says there is nothing wrong with the child, parents should explain what is happening on school days and ask for a referral to a child and adolescent psychiatrist or a child clinical psychologist. (If unsure whether it is school phobia, an educational psychologist can assess the child first.) A mental health professional experienced in dealing with children, adolescents and families is best able to help, may be able to spot other associated psychiatric disorders and will know the appropriate steps to take.

Other help and support may be obtained from a social worker, the educational welfare officer and the school psychologist; they can act as a link between parents and the school should problems arise. They may be able to make suggestions to the teachers on how best to handle the child and deal with her anxieties.

The child and adolescent psychiatrist

This person is a qualified medical doctor and fully trained psychiatrist who has additional training (beyond general psychiatry) with children, adolescents and families. The training of consultant child and adolescent psychiatrists includes approximately three years working in adult mental health services and other psychiatric sub-specialities, and three or more years specialising in work with children, young people and their families. They deal with a wide range of emotional and behavioural problems that both trouble children and worry those who care for them.

The child and adolescent psychiatrist tries to identify the problem and its cause and gives suggestions on how to help, using the knowledge he or she has of the family and school, the family's circumstances and the environment in which the child lives. He or she is also in touch with the child's school and doctor (with the parents' and child's agreement). Sometimes, medication is prescribed. Usually the child is helped as an outpatient in a hospital clinic. Most child and adolescent psychiatrists work within a multi-disciplinary team, which forms part of the local specialist Child and Adolescent Mental Health Service (CAMHS).

The psychologist

This person has a degree in psychology and may then specialise in clinical or educational psychology (taking at least six years in all). Psychologists can provide evaluation and treatment for emotional and behavioural problems and disorders, and can also provide testing and assessments. Educational psychologists have training and experience as teachers before specialising in educational psychology.

Psychologists work with individual children, families and groups of children and their parents, and can advise schools on how best to help the child. The child can be referred by the child's doctor to see a clinical psychologist, or parents can find a psychologist privately. The child's school can refer her to an educational psychologist, or parents can contact their local education authority direct.

The social worker

Social workers have a degree and some can provide forms of psycho-therapy such as family therapy or individual counselling (as can psychia-trists, psychologists, mental health nurses and psychotherapists), if they have had additional training.

Counsellors, therapists and psychotherapists

Parents may decide to pay for help privately from counsellors, therapists and psychotherapists if their child's difficulties are of long duration while waiting for an NHS referral. For difficulties of short duration, a referral may only take a month as these children tend to be prioritised.

Recovery is more likely with younger children, with children whose symptoms are less severe and with children who receive professional help early on. Some children will go on to have further emotional diffi-culties later in life.

Therapy for anxiety disorders

In general, a multi-pronged approach to treatment for a child with an anxiety disorder is likely to give a better result. Parents need to under-stand anxiety and what causes the child's symptoms and fears, in order to be supportive and help educate the child about the nature of her problem. A number of therapies are outlined below. I have given most weight to cognitive behavioural therapy, as I feel this can be very effec-tive in treating anxiety disorders and I had unwittingly used techniques from cognitive and behavioural therapies when helping my daughter.

Cognitive behavioural therapy

Cognitive behavioural therapy (CBT) combines two very effective kinds of psychotherapy: cognitive therapy and behavioural therapy.

The way the child feels about something (such as going to school) cannot be changed directly. One can't simply say to a child, 'You don't like school. I want you to like it' and then expect this to work. Indirect methods have to be used that are a combination of cognitive techniques (related to the thoughts the child has and how she perceives the world around her) that gradually change the child's thinking, and behavioural techniques.

The cognitive part of CBT is altering the child's ways of thinking for the better (correcting inaccurate or distorted views about herself and the world around her) and teaching the child how her thinking patterns are causing her symptoms. The behavioural part of CBT is helping the child to do things that will have a desirable effect on her life.

In CBT, the child will learn what she has to do to overcome her problems, and the changes she will have to make both in the way she thinks and feels and in the way she behaves and allows others to behave. CBT focuses on making a positive change in the child's life instead of just explaining why she has problems. For example, a child who does not interact with others or fails to make eye contact or smile will suggest to herself that no one likes her. She won't necessarily connect that it is due to her behaviour that others behave coolly towards her, because she hasn't made it easy for them to show that they do like her, or been prepared to open herself up to potential offers of friendship. The child needs to recognise that she is not inviting friendly overtures and can prove that this is the root of the problem by seeing what happens when she changes her behaviour and tries to become more sociable.

Usually CBT is carried out without the use of medication as it has been found to be very effective on its own. But if the child is unable to start treatment because of severe anxiety or because the treatment is hampered by severe anxiety (such as the child having repeated panic attacks, as in panic disorder), drugs may be used as well. However, they are always prescribed with caution because of the risks of addiction, dependence or toxicity. If drugs alone are used, without CBT, a relapse when the drugs are stopped is more likely because they have not helped the child learn valuable coping and emotional management skills. Other problems CBT can help with include:

- anxiety or worry

- depression and mood swings

- low self-esteem

- obsessive compulsive disorder

- panic attacks

- phobias

- post-traumatic stress

- school difficulties

- shyness and social anxiety.

CBT is a problem-oriented therapy during which the child's current difficulties are looked at in detail, to seek ways in which to deal with them, and which involves close collaboration between the child and therapist. The therapist and the child formulate the problem and set goals to work towards, with rewards to help motivate the child. The child is taught how to manage her anxiety and cope with her difficulties through a variety of techniques, including: monitoring her thoughts, feelings and behaviour; challenging her negative thoughts and beliefs; learning how her thoughts and feelings can affect the way her body feels; exposing her to the stressor in small steps, known as graduated exposure (desensitisation); role-playing; rewarding her verbally and materially for progress made; and learning relaxation skills.

Cognitive therapy

With cognitive therapy, the way the child's thoughts affect her feelings and behaviour is looked at. For example, if the child has told herself she should be afraid of school, she will feel scared and have bodily symptoms of fear when going to school, and her behaviour because of this fear might be one of avoidance.

Cognitive therapy is a way of helping children cope with stress and emotional problems. The child needs to understand that the way she feels about certain thoughts she has, about certain things that have happened to her and about how she views her world or how she thinks others see her, affects her emotionally and that these emotions can affect the way her body feels. For example, if the child is looking forward to something she will feel excited and this has an effect on her body, as do anxiety and fear. The child's emotions change her body's physiology by producing different hormones and neuro-chemicals which affect her bodily reactions.

If the child has learnt always to think and expect the worst, then she will continue to suffer unless her mind is trained or conditioned to think and respond differently to how it has in the past. Cognitive therapy assumes that if the child has become conditioned to think and feel negatively, then she can be reconditioned to think and feel more positively and rationally.

Cognitive therapy is probably not useful in very young children as they cannot identify the frightening or negative thoughts that they have, but therapists and parents could perhaps imagine what those thoughts are and supply different ways of viewing them. (This is what I did with my daughter: she learnt to 'self-talk' before she was seven years old.) Or, if the child has a theory that is distorted (such as 'The bus makes me vomit'), the therapist may be able to think of a way to put this to the test in order to disprove it to the child: 'Has it always made you vomit? Does it make all the children vomit or just you? How can it make only you vomit? That doesn't make sense. Perhaps it's something else that makes you vomit...'

With older children who can identify distressing thoughts, cognitive therapy helps them to assess these. Are their thoughts realistic? What would they think if a friend told them that was the way he saw it? What other viewpoints are there? Can they recognise that they have distorted their view of the situation and that this is why they feel badly about it?

The therapist can explain that unrealistic or distorted thoughts can undermine self-confidence and make the child feel depressed and anxious. Learning to look at these thoughts and beliefs in a different way can help the child cope better with life. These skills, once learnt, can be applied throughout the child's life, as the methods are the same for any problem. Once the child thinks more realistically, she will feel better and her symptoms will start to subside.

An example of using cognitive therapy for school phobia is when the child sees school as a frightening place. The thought of going to school makes her feel scared and she has bodily symptoms that tell her she is afraid. The child must look at her fear logically. If she's the only one who finds school scary (and she's not being bullied), it is unlikely that school really is scary; it's not a realistic thought. So the child could think of school as a neutral place that has potential for fun as well as learning; but she will have to look for that potential and recognise it. Knowing that in reality school is not a frightening place (that the child's thoughts are what's frightening her, not the school) can then lead to the child 'knowing' that it is a safe place, that she can look for positive things the school has to offer and that this will help her think of it in a positive light and lessen her anxiety about going (see Chapter Six on using charts).

The therapist is not likely to give the child all the answers; an important part of cognitive therapy is for the child to work these out herself, because then she can do it on her own throughout her life – she has been given a vital life skill that allows her to question her own behaviour and thoughts as well as others'. However, the therapist can put forward suggestions.

An example of how a child can use cognitive therapy at a later date would be when the child has been ill and off school and has lost confidence about going back. She may feel ill after her parents have pronounced her well, and be convinced that if she were to return to school she would be ill there. If she can recognise the symptoms as possibly being anxiety symptoms (different to when she was ill), she can then ask herself if she was actually anxious. To test this she can reflect on what her thoughts and feelings were, regarding returning to school. If she can recognise that she was dreading the return and didn't feel safe about going back, she can reassure herself that the best thing for her is to go back and get on with it. (This will have been proven in the past and she can remember this too.)

Cognitive therapy is about problem solving: identifying all current problem areas of the child's life and then finding solutions.

The things I said to help my daughter

At the time, I did not know that the methods I used to help my daughter could be defined as cognitive or behavioural therapy. I said and did the things instinctively, thinking about how I rationalise my own problems and fears. The things outlined below were said to a young six-year-old, with positive effect. I personally believe that the key to any child's school phobia is through CBT, but with the parent being equally educated about this in relation to school phobia as a co-therapist. The parent is, after all, with the child much of the time and is actually present during the height of the child's distress, something that the therapist can't be.

If the child thinks the professional doesn't know what is happening to her, her stress will increase as she may think she's dying or that there's something dreadfully wrong with her that a visit to the specialist can't put right. Her previous experiences have been about going to the doctor and being told she has such and such. Sometimes she would have been given medicine and she'd soon have been better or she'd have been told that her illness would get better on its own, needing only a few days of rest.

Thus, to suddenly realise that there's no quick fix is probably very frightening. The child may have even been told that there is nothing wrong with her. But she knows there is, because otherwise she wouldn't feel so bad. She may think that the doctor has made a mistake and missed what the problem is and that she might die before her parents realise she's terribly ill. She needs to have her problem recognised (by sympathetic carers) and then calmly explained to her in simple terms.

The child should be told she has 'school phobia'. The relief of knowing the name of her problem and that many children have it might make a big difference to the child's mental attitude. She needs to feel she can beat it with help – not that it is a hopeless, unknown thing that has happened to her that no one can help her with.

Telling my own daughter that she had school phobia was late in coming – I did not know it was school phobia at the beginning and after that worried about labelling her with a mental health problem. But children do not have the prejudices and fears of stigma as adults do, and the absolute relief she experienced (noticed in the days following) of having a name for her condition made a huge difference. It was suddenly a confirmed diagnosis, something definite that she could work on to recover from. It also gave her the verbal skills to better talk about it. 'When will my school phobia go?' ('When you manage to relax and not worry about going to school.') Several years on, my daughter would occasionally say, 'When I had school phobia ...' It became a useful addition to our language at home.

It should be explained to the child why she feels the way she does in words she can understand: 'Your brain is frightening you with nasty thoughts that don't make sense. It needs to be taught that these thoughts aren't true, that it got it wrong.'

The child should be told that she feels ill because of worry: worrying makes her over-breathe, giving her unpleasant symptoms, and that when she is worried her body makes 'worry' hormones that also make her feel ill.

The 'vicious circle' also needs to be explained to the child. Therapists construct a formulation of the problem, along with the child and parents, to explain how it evolved and what is prolonging the problem. For example, in explaining my daughter's (agoraphobic) fears about going on the school bus, I said:

> When you stepped in dog poo and smelt it on the bus, you felt sick. When you were about to go on the bus the next time, your brain said to you, 'Hey, the last time you went on the bus, you felt sick. You'll feel sick this time too.' So you started to worry about feeling sick on the bus and this made you feel sick because you believed what your brain said to you.
>
> Then your brain said to you, 'You don't like going on the bus, it makes you feel sick – you might even be sick.' So you started to think you would be sick and felt even sicker. Your brain reminded you that you could be sick (because of when you went to hospital by ambulance and you kept vomiting) so you worried all the more and felt worse.
>
> By the time you had to get on the bus, you felt so sick you were convinced you would be and it frightened you. Your brain panicked and said, 'Don't get on the bus or you'll be sick. You know you will. You feel very sick already. It's getting worse, not better. Soon you will be sick.' You believed this and decided not to get on, but your dad forced you on. You spent the whole journey thinking about feeling sick and worrying that you might be. Your brain said, 'You see? I was right. It is worse now. You'll be sick soon.'
>
> You lasted the journey but you felt so ill by the time you got to school you still felt like you were going to be sick. You didn't know what was happening to you and it frightened you even more. You thought you must be very ill. And then you were sick.
>
> Your original problem, the dog poo, was not around any more, but you believed you still had a problem because of what your brain

told you. It started off as a little problem and grew into a big problem because your brain told you lies. It didn't understand that you felt sick on the bus because of the poo, but thought it was the bus or going to school that made you ill. It is not the bus or the school that makes you feel sick, it is worry. If you can stop these worrying thoughts, you will stop feeling sick.

Also, you thought that being sick was a serious illness as you had been sick before the ambulance came and during your ride in the ambulance. You may have thought that if you were sick on the bus or in school, you were ill enough to need an ambulance. But you know that just being sick is not serious. The reason you went to hospital was not because of your being sick but because you had croup. That can be a serious illness.

Understanding how anxiety works breaks the fear of not knowing why certain things are happening. Parents can use a similar explanation with a child who has difficulties, and she will soon self-talk and tell herself the same reassuring things. However, some children find self-talking harder than others.

If the child is vomiting from anxiety, her fear of being sick needs to be reduced. It could be pointed out that she has been sick a great many times. She is used to it. It isn't pleasant but it doesn't hurt her. She could be told, 'Accept that these feelings will be there and they will become boring to you. You know they'll be there and so you won't be surprised. Because you know they'll be there, you needn't worry about when exactly they do come. Just accept them. Then try to carry on as normal, without letting them upset you.

If you are sick, never mind. Do not try to fight it, let it come. You only get more worried if you do try to fight these feelings. When you are less worried and less upset by what happens, these feelings will start to go.

However, most children aren't ever sick from anxiety so such advice could increase their fear of being sick. Many children fear the anticipated public humiliation of being sick more than the event itself.

Some children soil themselves through anxiety because they get diarrhoea. Although this too is unpleasant, similar talk can help allay these fears. The key to it is stopping the child's negative thoughts and the resultant panic she experiences.

The child can be told:

> You know that school is not bad for you: you've been there loads of times without anything happening to you and everything's been fine. You've been on the bus many times too without anything happening to you. It is not these things that make you ill. The only difference now is that you have frightening thoughts about these things and your body is sensing danger because your mind is telling you lies and you believe them.

The child also needs to counteract the negative thoughts she has by having them challenged and swapping them with helpful thoughts. Giving her alternative thoughts in this way encourages her to positively self-talk. These helpful thoughts are valuable, as eventually they will stay in her mind and she can use them at any time she is anxious. Examples of positive alternatives are:

- This is a hard thing to beat, but with help I can.

- I know I'm not ill. I've had these feelings before and I recognise them as worry feelings.

- I don't like feeling like this but it won't hurt me.

- These feelings won't last for long.

- I need to get stuck into things and forget about how my body feels. Then these feelings will go away.

- If I ignore these feelings, they will not get worse and will gradually go.

- It's natural to have feelings like this when I am worried.

- Lots of other people feel like this too. We need to be brave.

- I have learnt to worry about these feelings and it has made them worse. Now I need to tell them that they don't matter and that I'm carrying on anyway.

- When my brain tells me things that frighten me I must tell it to STOP and think of something nice. (I can have a list of nice things to remember for when this happens.)

The child could be asked to estimate when she feels she has calmed down in school, and as a measure of her progress in therapy, every week or so she could be asked again. This can then be used as a marker to see how well the child is responding.

With my daughter, the marker shifted from the afternoon – I think lunchtime was stressful because she found it so hard to eat – to before first break until, finally, she felt calm as soon as she arrived in school. Therapists often use a scoring method, such as asking the child to keep a diary of how she feels each day, at various times through the day, on a scale of 1 to 10 (where 10 represents the most fearful and uncomfortable feelings and 1 the most relaxed and comfortable feelings the child has). Any improvements will be evident and the therapist can ask the child what helped her scores become closer to 1 on those occasions. This will help the child identify coping mechanisms she has been unconsciously using so that she can consciously learn to do more of the same; the diary will provide concrete evidence that the child is learning to deal with her difficulties so that she is motivated to persevere.

Once the child has identified the point when she's calm in school, she could be asked why it is that she feels better then. She could also be asked if there is anything during the school day that she does not like, in order to identify difficult areas. My daughter didn't like registration as she had once been sick from anxiety during it and found that registration wasn't sufficiently directed to distract her – she preferred being given work to do. It would have helped if the teacher had sat her down to work on arrival. The child may not know what has helped her settle, but suggestions could be made:

- Are you more relaxed because you have been given work to do?

- Do you like to be busy?

- Is there something you like doing?

- Do you like talking to the children you sit with?

- Is there something in the day that you don't look forward to and you're glad when it's over?

Once what it is that helps the child to settle has been identified, what she could do to help herself settle earlier could be discussed. Basically, the key to getting a child out of an intense anxiety state is distraction and interest in things outside herself. On the way to school, she could make conversation or try to notice the weather, the trees and plants she passes, any major landmarks, the cars that pass, any pets she sees and so on. This may only help once the child has started to recover, but the theory is useful.

The first day of school in the September after my daughter had started to recover from school phobia (she was still only six) brought anxiety and a stomachache. But without prompting she said to me, 'I expect it will go when I get to school,' and it did. She had learnt and remembered that the best thing for her was to get stuck in. She has said similar things about school since, and about other things she's been nervous about. If she's nervous, I remind her she'll be fine once there and because she has learnt this is true, she believes it and is fine.

Behavioural therapy

Most of the child's behaviour is learned, even when it is related to, and influenced by, her genes. Unhelpful behaviour is a result of defective learning. Behavioural therapy focuses on the child's current obvious behaviour problems (such as avoidance) and teaches her to respond to things in a different way, through rewarding her for positive actions and positive behaviour changes. Behavioural therapy can include learning relaxation techniques and desensitisation (by gradually increasing the child's exposure to the stressful event or thing).

POSITIVE BEHAVIOUR CHANGES: CONDITIONING

If something happens that makes the child react with fear or anxiety, her consequent actions will affect how she thinks in the future. For example, if she felt ill on the bus and got off, she may think that it was because she got off that she stopped feeling ill and that it was the bus that made her ill. She will then want to protect herself from feeling ill again and will tell herself that she must avoid getting on the bus. Getting off has taught her that avoidance is necessary, and feeling fine after getting off the bus reinforces the false learning.

So the child's thinking, under the influence of an automatic emotional reaction, becomes unhelpful. Sometimes parents unwittingly reinforce school phobia by allowing the child to stay at home rather than confront her fears. However, this should not be seen as apportioning blame. It is natural for parents to comply with their child when she is in great distress, begging them not to make her go to school. They are programmed to gather the child to them and fuss over her. And if the child is severely affected, this may be the kindest and least harmful option for her until she receives appropriate professional help.

Much of behaviour therapy derives from Pavlov's dog, who was conditioned to expect food when he heard a buzzer because he had regularly been fed when the buzzer sounded. The dog salivated at the sound of the buzzer without seeing or smelling the food, because the expectation was there. He hadn't previously thought that the sound of a buzzer would indicate the arrival of food but because this kept happening, he learnt that the buzzer meant food was coming.

But when Pavlov used the buzzer too often without producing food, the dog no longer salivated just because of the sound. So Pavlov concluded that a conditioned reaction could be overridden if it was no longer reinforced.

This can be related to children who are afraid of going to school. If they are made to go to school often enough (or travel on the bus) and find that nothing bad happens to them, eventually their false conditioning should be overridden because they experience that school is not such a threatening place. However, it may be helpful for the child to first understand that it is her thoughts that have been making her feel ill, as there is a risk that unsuccessful reconditioning attempts might further confirm the false conditioning.

I made up a desensitisation programme (see *Desensitisation* below) that my daughter agreed to follow, to help her get back on the school bus, as I had been driving her to school for some weeks. (She managed to come home on the bus each day without much difficulty.) Although the idea terrified her at first, after a week or so of reminding her that it was not the bus that made her feel ill but the thought of going to school and worrying about being ill there, she agreed. In this way she was successfully reconditioned (it did take a few weeks) to go back on the bus without being sick and managed to return to full-time attendance (previously three-days-a-week attendance had been agreed with her doctor and the educational welfare officer, on health grounds).

Children more readily adopt behaviour that is rewarded so they need to have goals and rewards to motivate them (but this does not work the opposite way: children *should not* be punished for non-useful behaviour). Thus, the therapist could work out with the child's parents what rewards would be appropriate for the child having to put herself through a painful reconditioning in order to regain a normal life. And it is not only the child's parents who need to engage in this: the child's teachers also need to be part of the reward process. They must not say or do anything to show disapproval; they must show understanding and give lavish praise when the child has made a step, however small, in the right direction.

POSITIVE BEHAVIOUR CHANGES: MODELLING

Behavioural therapy also includes taking positive action that does not necessarily have anything to do with *re*conditioning. For example, if a child is very shy and socially anxious, the therapist can work at ways to help the child's social skills and can role-play situations to make her feel confident about them in real life situations (details of social skills training books are given at the end of Chapter Five).

The child can be taught how to observe others' behaviour: what they say, how they say it and what they do, and then copy it in her own way. This is called modelling (or imitating). It is very useful for children who need to develop their social skills. The child needs to watch and pay attention to the behaviour she witnesses, remember what she has seen, reproduce the behaviour herself and be motivated by being rewarded. Positively reinforcing her skilful behaviour will help condition the child into using it.

An example of modelling in the treatment of selective mutism (see Chapter Five) is for the child to watch, when in the company of the therapist, a video of herself talking at home, to encourage her to speak in the presence of the therapist. Here the child is modelling herself. However, selectively mute children often become silent if they are aware of the presence of a video recorder, so this may not be possible.

With my own daughter, her anxiety had made her behaviour change towards other people *before school*. She would ignore everyone, including her peers at the bus stop, would not show any interest in the conversation around her, and would not make eye contact or smile a greeting. When I was starting the desensitisation programme of getting her back on the school bus after her break, I pointed out to her how her behaviour had changed and asked her to remember that she used to talk to her friends and look pleased to see them. I wanted her to model herself on how she had been (to become reconditioned to behaving as she used to). I also told her that there was no point in my travelling on the bus with her after the initial day or two, because the way forward was for her to be with her friends and interact with them, and my presence interfered with that. Pointing out to her how she had changed her behaviour, and how this was affecting her time with her friends in the mornings, helped.

Relaxation techniques

Relaxation techniques train the child to 'listen' to her body and to notice when it is tense. She can then carry out muscle tensing and relaxing to help calm her and recall calming thoughts. She can also perform relaxation exercises at bedtime to help her sleep and give her a more relaxing sleep. Listening to calming music may also help. This is dealt with more thoroughly in *Using relaxation techniques* in Chapter Five. Suggestions of relaxation cassettes/CDs are given in *Further Resources*. Relaxation can also help increase the child's self-esteem and give her positive thoughts, as her mind is more receptive when relaxed. She can imagine herself as the confident and happy child she'd like to be.

Children can also be desensitised to anxiety-provoking events by imagining them when in a relaxed state (see *Desensitisation* below). When children are thoroughly distracted, it gives their minds and bodies a break from the adrenaline and hyperventilation that cause their unpleasant symptoms. The suggestions below can help a child who is too young to learn relaxation techniques or to add an extra dimension to work with those who can.

Distraction

Parents could deliberately try having sufficient time before school for the child to do a regular activity to distract her completely so that her anxiety symptoms become reduced. This may limit the height her anxiety reaches when it's time to leave for school (although the child probably needs to be partially recovered to be able to focus on these). Suggestions for such activities are:

- practising a musical instrument (because music lessons and instruments are expensive, the child will need to have wanted to learn anyway, and parents need to have the financial resources)

- playing a demanding computer game

- completing a maths puzzle

- building a complicated Lego structure (from plans)

- completing a very hard jigsaw puzzle.

Watching television may be too passive for very anxious children, although it may distract only mildly affected children.

The child needs to enjoy the activity to be motivated to stick with it, or she may need parental involvement to help her settle to it. The activity might be more successful if it is only carried out before school (also motivating the child to get ready quickly to have time for it). Or it could be started the night before to give the child something to look forward to for the next morning and, each time a new project is started, it could be begun in the evening with the need to carry on in the morning.

For all the activities except practising a musical instrument, the child could have relaxing music in the background to listen to, which would occupy more of her mind and have a calming effect of its own.

Using behaviour to increase the child's self-esteem

Children who are fit and enjoy playing physical games and playing a musical instrument (or dancing) are more likely to feel better about themselves and have a high self-esteem. Such activities should be encouraged. Being physically active can also counteract the child's feelings of anxiety.

Desensitisation

Desensitisation involves the child putting herself in a stressful situation and becoming so used to it that her previous bodily sensations of fear and anxiety fade because she has done it so often. Desensitisation that is done in a complete way rather than building up in little steps to the stressful event is known as 'flooding'. An example of flooding is leaving a highly school phobic child in school after she has had time off and is unable to contemplate attending. This can be very hard for the child and could cause great distress. Gradual desensitisation (also known as graduated exposure) is kinder and is less likely to traumatise the child. (Flooding is now rarely used as a therapy technique and usually only with consenting adults.)

An example of gradual desensitisation for a school phobic child (suffering from agoraphobia) is getting the child to watch the other children arrive at school for one week, then having to stand in the schoolyard for five minutes another week, building up to ten minutes, then attending school for registration and so on until, finally, one school day is completed. The child should be praised and rewarded for every tiny achievement, and backward steps should not be punished.

Desensitisation can also be used with relaxation techniques so that, while the child is completely relaxed, things that make her anxious are talked about or watched, or the therapist describes a situation. As the child copes with each scene or situation, she is given progressively more difficult ones to cope with until she no longer feels anxious about, for example, going to school.

A selectively mute child (see Chapter Five) can also be helped using desensitisation while relaxed. She imagines talking to different people, on a scale of increasing difficulty, while in a relaxed state. (She can choose the order of the people she will imagine talking to.) Then the child can try talking to these people in real life, having previously chosen suitable rewards for each step.

However, the selectively mute child can work on a desensitisation programme without relaxed visualisation. If the child is happy to talk to her parent, she can try as the next step to talk to someone else whom she regards as the next least threatening person while in her parent's company. And then she can progress to another person. Later she might be able to talk to new people without the company of her parent, but with someone else she has learnt to talk to earlier in the desensitisation programme. Eventually, the child will be able to talk to everyone she needs to.

However, with desensitisation it should be stressed that the child should not be forced to progress at a rate at which she feels uncomfortable. If the child has problems at a particular stage, she should learn to cope at that level before moving on.

DESENSITISATION PROGRAMME USED WITH MY DAUGHTER TO GET HER BACK ON THE SCHOOL BUS

Before this programme could be effected I had had long chats with my daughter and had reasoned with her, as described in *Cognitive therapy* above. I had also taught her to empty her own vomit down the toilet at school, rinse out her little bucket, throw the rinsing water down the toilet and then to tie the bucket up in a plastic bag to bring it home in a clean way. She was also given a drink to have after she'd vomited. She was little more than six when she learnt to do this, but was quite capable of it. No one at school offered to help her on arrival, so she had to do it on her own if she were not to have me with her all the time, which would have been counter-productive.

I also talked matter-of-factly about the whole process: I showed confidence in my daughter and in the programme, without giving signs of worrying about her. I cheerfully said goodbye, gave her a big kiss and cuddle, and then left. This was very hard to do but I knew it must be done. This is the programme I used:

1. Travel on the bus with me sitting next to you.

2. Travel on the bus with me sitting behind you. (This was important because my daughter had stopped communicating with anyone else before school. She needed to get back to socialising with her friends and my sitting next to her did not help that.)

3. Travel on the bus alone. I'll see you onto it and then meet the bus and see you into school. (These steps worked like

magic until about the third day when she was so happy getting off the bus, she ignored me and walked into school chatting with friends. I thought I should go straight home and did. I found out she'd been sick in school because I hadn't carried on the ritual she demanded, of going with her to the cloakroom and waiting for her to go to the toilet before saying goodbye. The next day she vomited in her little bucket on the bus, which made her friend move seats because of the smell. I had just started breakfast with her in the mornings as the programme had been going so well, so had to revert to breakfast in school at first break. I also quickly moved on to the next stage as my daughter had regressed on this one and the stress of saying goodbye twice was not helping.)

4. Travel on the bus alone. (I said goodbye to her and left it at that.)

My daughter was only occasionally sick after this until the vomiting stopped altogether (about six weeks later). Her anxiety was still present and life was tough for her, but it was so much better.

I had told her I was angry when she'd complained that I hadn't joined her in school on the day she'd been so happy in step three (but had later vomited). Instead of allowing her to go back a step, I moved her on, as I felt she was capable of going it alone. I also suspected her of using the situation to prove to me she still needed me there, but we both needed more independence. Logically, she knew that nothing could happen to her.

The parent must be prepared to keep stepping back. With the right support, children can cope with more than we can imagine and I told my daughter how proud I was of her for being so brave: because what she was doing was the bravest thing she'd ever done, despite it being a simple matter to her peers.

OTHER BEHAVIOURAL CONSIDERATIONS WITH MY DAUGHTER

The school bus programme was not used in isolation to what was going on in the rest of my daughter's life. There was another family who regularly invited my daughter out with theirs on trips. I'd dose my daughter with a travel sickness pill and cheerfully say goodbye to her and her friend. The friend's parents were happy to deal with whatever happened and my daughter never refused to go with them. Nor was she ever sick when with them: vomiting was confined to school days. They accepted her numerous trips to the toilet and never criticised her, which was why my daughter continued to feel at ease with them. Their help was a major factor in my daughter's recovery.

I never physically forced her to go anywhere she didn't want to (except for the one time my husband carried her on to the school bus, before we knew what was up). She accepted that school was a must and on the days she didn't go to school during her part-time attendance, I gave her school-type work in the mornings (provided by myself as the school didn't allow any books home apart from a reading book) and kept to the timing of the start of school, morning break and lunchtimes. In the afternoons she was free to play and watch videos. After school she had a friend come round.

AN EXAMPLE OF USING COGNITIVE BEHAVIOURAL THERAPY TO FACILITATE A POSITIVE CHANGE IN THE CHILD

If the child sees school as an unfriendly place that makes her feel unwelcome, the child could be asked why she thinks school is unfriendly (the cognitive part). Seeing school as an unfriendly place might be true if the child has no friends. Does she really have no friends? If she doesn't, why not? Do friends come automatically or is there something she has to do to show that she's interested in others? How does she think they see her? (They probably see her as unfriendly and uninterested, because she doesn't smile at them, keeps herself to herself and doesn't ask to join in.)

The child can then make behavioural changes such as initiating conversation with a peer, asking to join in games and smiling at people. This will reap the reward of her feeling socially included, which will then lead her to make further behavioural changes. My book, *Social Awareness Skills for Children*, mentioned at the end of Chapter Five, is full of role-plays and examples to use for social interactions in a variety of settings that could help the child respond more positively to others and make friends.

Family therapy

Family therapy is based on the idea that emotional and behavioural difficulties in children, such as separation anxiety, affect the whole family and that the family is needed to help solve the child's problems. Some family therapists may see the child in individual sessions and use the outcome of these in a later family session. Support from a family therapist may include helping the child to face new situations rather than withdrawing from them, and helping families to change the way they act towards each other.

Sometimes family therapists work with one-way mirrors, with other therapists watching from an adjoining room, to better understand the family's interactions. The therapists in the adjoining room can, for example, make suggestions to the therapist in the room via a telephone, without making the child more anxious by having several people in the same room. It also means that the family deal with one therapist only, instead of several, increasing the opportunity to build trust and collaboration.

The family is often very much needed in helping the distressed child. For example, the family can reinforce what the therapist says, repeat the expressions the therapist uses to explain the child's problems and provide opportunities for the child to increase her social interactions by inviting friends and other people to the home.

There are many forms of family therapy. Below, mention has been made of systemic family therapy,[*] solution focused brief therapy and motivational interviewing.

SYSTEMIC FAMILY THERAPY

Systemic family therapy looks at the systems that affect the child, including the systems working within the family (child members, the family as a unit, the extended family) and wider systems such as social services and schools, as they all have an effect on the child. It also

---

[*]   The terms 'systems' and 'systemic' have also been claimed by many other family therapy models, for example, Milan systemic (Selvini et al. 1980), strategic (Haley 1973), structural (Minuchin 1974), narrative (White and Epston 1990) and solution focused approaches (de Shazer 1982).

requires an awareness of the effect of the therapist and the therapist's team, on the child's systems, for example, previous professional and personal experiences (so-called 'second order' family therapy).

Systemic family therapy operates from a neutral, non-blaming position (looking at the family as a whole, without casting blame on an individual) and respects cultural, race, gender, sexual orientation and lifestyle differences. If the therapist is unfamiliar with the clients' culture, for example, he or she asks questions to aid understanding.

All members of the family invited to sessions have an opportunity to say how they feel about things that have happened and how they feel about each other, while being supported by the therapist, so that the sessions are constructive rather than destructive. During this time, the therapist will identify and explore the family's thoughts, beliefs, myths or attitudes, which may be contributing to the child's difficulties.

The therapist may also explore those solutions the family have already tried and will amplify any positive changes to the child, so that she is motivated to do more of the same and look for further solutions (systemic therapy may use techniques from solution focused brief therapy, outlined below). This should lead to the child and family members feeling that they have the problem under control.

SOLUTION FOCUSED BRIEF THERAPY

Solution focused brief therapy (SFBT) and the related solution oriented brief therapy (also called possibility therapy) take up as few sessions as possible. Therapists seek to find solutions to problems that exist in the present and SFBT is very much goal-oriented with the child, her family and the therapist working together to find solutions. The child and family work collaboratively with the therapist to achieve the goals the child wants.

One of the core beliefs of SFBT is that the family has all the resources it needs at its disposal to solve its problems. It focuses on strengths and abilities rather than weaknesses, and looks for exceptions to the problem to supply a solution (for example, how the child coped before the difficulty arose or how she has managed similar difficulties in the past). Understanding how these occasions alleviated the problem helps the child and family recreate them. If an exception can't be thought of, the therapist will make suggestions of things to try. The child's teachers can help the child and therapist find solutions by noting when the child's difficulty is less or absent, or what makes the child's difficulties worse. This will give information on what things should be avoided and what things can be changed, to bring about further lessening or an absence of the child's difficulties. The child's teachers can also provide positive comments about the child's strengths and skills so that she sees herself as a capable person and not one who is a failure. The child can then remind herself of her positive qualities and work on improving these, which may have a positive effect on her difficulties.

The therapist may ask the child questions such as, 'How do you make your problem easier to manage?' or 'What things do you say to yourself to help you through the hard times?' or 'How have you stopped your problem from getting worse?' or 'When is your problem less of a problem? Why do you think that is?' or 'You say you've had a similar problem before. What did you do to make things better then?' These identify the coping skills the child already has, so that they can be consciously used by her to greater effect and to show the child that she already has the strengths and skills to deal with her difficulties.

MOTIVATIONAL INTERVIEWING

Some adolescents in distress develop risky behaviour in an effort to deal with their anxiety. Motivational interviewing (MI) techniques can be used to help those who have, for example, eating disorders or alcohol, tobacco or drug habits, or those who indulge in risky sexual activity, to become motivated about changing their habits or behaviour when they are ambivalent (feeling two ways about it) or resistant to change.

The techniques used in MI help the adolescent discover her own reasons for change, to create internal conflict so that she can reflect upon present behaviour and personal goals. The therapist needs to understand from the adolescent's perspective in order to identify her personal goals and the priorities and concerns she has in life, so topics of discussion can be wide-ranging. MI is respectful of the adolescent, acknowledges the choices facing her and accepts her ambivalence to change, without increasing resistance to it at a time when she may be naturally pushing against authority and trying to find her own identity and place in the world. Techniques used in MI include:

- Expressing empathy (showing the child that the therapist understands the child's difficulties from her perspective and that the therapist accepts the child as she is without showing that he or she wants her to change)

- Reflective listening (repeating back phrases the child uses to show that the therapist is listening carefully, or summing up something the child has said so the therapist can check that he or she understands what the child has said or wants to say)

- Asking open-ended questions (questions where the therapist does not show an expectation of a yes-no answer, or those that have only a small number of defined answers such as when asking the child, did you feel this or that?)

- Being supportive to the child and showing her that she is doing all right (affirming); this can be done, for example, by agreeing with something the child says, sympathising with her over something that must have been hard for her to cope with and making positive comments about the child

- Asking questions that promote talking about the need to change, such as asking about the disadvantages of how things are now, the advantages the child may experience if she were to change, the personal strengths the child has that can help her change and what things the child would be willing to try.

MI is not about the therapist taking a superior role as one who knows what is best for the child or about pressurising the child to change. The therapist will ensure that his or her role is a supportive and interested one, where he or she works collaboratively with the child to help her work out the priorities she has stemming from her own values, and how things can be done differently to help her reach her personal goals.

Once the child has been motivated to change, she will be more open to other forms of therapy to help with underlying problems and may be more ready to make a commitment to securing that change.

Drug treatments for anxiety disorders

Drug treatments for anxiety disorders would be used as a last resort by an experienced professional when the non-medical treatments were proven to be ineffective and the child's life was severely affected, such as being unable to go to school at all. They would also be used for a severely affected child who is too anxious to respond to therapy because, for example, she is having frequent panic attacks or suffering panic disorder. Drugs can stop panic attacks and relieve a child's depression. There are side effects, however, but none of the drugs used for children should have side effects that continue after the drug has been stopped.

When drugs are prescribed for children, the starting dose is usually lower than it is for adults, depending on the age and size of the child. The prescribing professional may slowly increase the dose to reduce unpleasant side effects, until there is an improvement in the child's mental health. The child may be monitored for weight changes, tics (involuntary movements or vocal sounds), depression, mania, blood pressure and pulse rate; she may also need blood tests. However, for most drugs used with children this will be unnecessary.

There has been less research into drug treatments for children and adolescents with anxiety-related problems than with adults because of the difficulties drug companies have in getting ethics approval for trials with these age groups. This issue is now being addressed as companies are being financially encouraged to undertake clinical trials with children.

Psychotropic medications that are used to treat anxiety disorders in children fall into two groups – anti-depressants and benzodiazepines.

Anti-depressants

Not all anxiolytic (anxiety-reducing) anti-depressants are effective for the same conditions. Choice of which anti-depressant to use is based on how effective a drug is for a particular condition, whether there are coexisting conditions (that make a particular drug efficacious for both, for example) and the side effects it may have.

SELECTIVE SEROTONIN REUPTAKE INHIBITORS (SSRIs)

Selective serotonin reuptake inhibitors work by regulating mood, appetite, sleep, aggression, and obsessions and compulsions. They include citalopram (Cipramil), fluvoxamine (Faverin), paroxetine (Seroxat), fluoxetine (Prozac) and sertraline (Lustral), and are useful in the treatment of depression, anxiety, panic and obsessive compulsive disorders. They are generally well tolerated, the side effects including stomach upset, insomnia or drowsiness, and headaches. In rare cases these drugs can make the child stiff and have unusual movements, but these disappear after a few months of use (however, the child may not experience all or any of these).

It may take six to eight weeks before the effects of this type of drug become apparent and up to three months before the full effect is seen. If one drug does not suit a child, another in the same group might. It is a case of trial and error and much patience is needed. The effects of the drug may take longer to appear since the doses have to be initially very low; sometimes these drugs can make the child more anxious to begin with.

When taking a SSRI, parents need to be careful that the child is not prescribed any other medication with which it may adversely interact.

TRICYCLIC ANTI-DEPRESSANTS

Tricyclic anti-depressants are not usually used for childhood or adolescent depression as there is no evidence that they work with this age group. However, amitriptyline (Lentizol) may occasionally be used for chronic pain such as trigeminal neuralgia. Clomipramine (Anafranil) is used in treating obsessive compulsive disorder and imipramine (Tofranil) in bedwetting (although the child will need to be monitored with electro-cardiograms every three months unless the drug is given in slowly increasing doses; also, having it in the house poses a danger to younger siblings because of the risk of overdose).

The side effects of tricyclic anti-depressants are: blurry vision, constipation, drowsiness, dry mouth, headache, orthostatic hypotension (low blood pressure when standing still), stomach upset, urinary retention, agitation and sweating (however, the child may not experience all or any of these).

OTHER ANTI-DEPRESSANTS

Venlafaxine (Effexor), mirtazapine (Remeron) and nefazodone (Serzone) are new medications considered for use in anxiety and depression, but there is little data regarding their use with children. The side effects include hypertension (high blood pressure), sleep disturbance and stomach upset (however, the child may not experience all or any of these).

Benzodiazepines

Benzodiazepines are rarely prescribed to children in the UK and usually only for short-term use. These drugs are tranquillisers that calm the mind. There is a possibility of addiction with these drugs, although those that work more quickly are more addictive than those that have a slow build-up. Also, those that leave the bloodstream quickly have an increased likelihood of causing addiction. For example, Chlordiazepoxide (Librium), goes in and out of the body's system slowly. Diazepam (Valium), however, goes in fast and comes out slowly, so has a moderate addiction risk. The use of benzodiazepines in the management of child and adolescent anxiety remains poorly studied and understood.

Rethinking school

Since attending school is so stressful for the child (and so for the rest of the family), parents may need to rethink whether this is the right place for her. Parents may need to ask themselves:

- Is this the right school for the child?

- Are teachers treating her appropriately?

- Is the child unable to cope with large-scale mainstream education? The move from primary to secondary school can be very daunting, particularly for those children who have been schooled in rural areas with very small primary schools.

- Are there special units within the school that can offer accommodation to a child who has special needs because of her anxieties?

- Should the child change school? If so, would it be to another state school or to a private school (for example)? If parents decide to change the child's school, it is vital they meet with the headteacher, spend time in the school and have the child spend time there too. What are the benefits of this new school? What are the downsides? (For example, are the children pressurised to do well? This would not suit a school phobic child.)

Generally, professional advice is never to withdraw the child from school. Professionals feel this is a big mistake and that it makes it all the harder to reintegrate the child into the school environment. Often it is a period of absence in the first place that has triggered school phobia, so more of the same is not likely to improve it.

However, if the child's school phobia does not improve even after several weeks of forcing her to go to school, and perhaps worsens, or the child refuses attendance altogether and is too old to be forced, parents may decide to go ahead with school withdrawal (see *Home education* below). Without the appropriate help, understanding and support, forcing a severely affected child to attend school can both traumatise her and damage her emotionally, giving her further problems in the future.

Withdrawing the child from school is a very difficult decision for parents to make; partners may differ in their views and may not be supported by significant others in their lives such as friends, parents and parents-in-law, and the child's teachers. A child can be withdrawn from school:

- temporarily, with the expectation of returning as soon as she has received professional help, in very small stages to desensitise her to the school environment. Done at the child's pace, with some pressure to move forwards, the child can gradually accept that school is not such a hostile environment as previously supposed (unless bullying is involved, in which case this would have to be dealt with first; see Chapter Three: Bullying)

- part-time as in my daughter's case; she returned to school full-time as soon as she could cope (albeit with some effort)

- for a year or two and educated at home

- permanently and educated at home; but many parents simply do not have this as an option.

However, the longer the child is out of school, the harder it is for her to return. Also, her social development may be affected while she is not in a school environment. If parents decide to go down this road, they will first need to thoroughly research what the consequences are and what they will need to do to fulfil the child's educational needs and satisfy the local education authority. (Parents can find this out by contacting a home education group, details of which are given in *Useful Contacts* at the end of this book.) Or they might want to apply to their local education authority for home tuition via the child's school. It is easier for parents to obtain home tuition if a medical recommendation is given that suggests that the child's difficulties preventing her from attending school are medical in nature, for example, where there is a diagnosis of anxiety or depression.

Older children may be able to enrol early at a further education college, as they may feel more comfortable in an environment where the structure is not so rigid.

Parents may feel they must home educate a severely affected child, either because they see it as the only option or because they are not willing for the child to be put through further turmoil (risking further psychiatric problems) and want the child's distress to end immediately. Children who suffer from autistic spectrum disorders may experience high levels of anxiety anyway and can often develop other conditions (such as depression and obsessive compulsive disorders and other phobias) as a result of chronic and intense anxiety. This means that they need to be rescued from an environment that is not helping them, either temporarily or permanently (see *Special schools for children with autistic spectrum disorders* in Chapter One).

Home education

If a child's poor attendance or non-attendance at school is due to severe anxieties, the educational welfare department needs to become involved. An educational welfare officer can advise parents on what they must do and what their rights are, and give them information on home education.

The local education authority may provide home tuition if the parent wishes the child eventually to go back into full-time mainstream education: the home tuition service is regarded as a temporary reintegration service. The tuition may be provided in the child's home (although with school phobia, this may make a child even more dependent on the home environment), in a small group held at a centre or a combination of the two. Home tuition is often for a maximum of two and a half hours per day when provided in a school unit and often far less when provided at home.

Should parents feel that they want a permanent (or long-term) break from mainstream schooling for the child, they will need to prove that they are educating her appropriately at home. One way of doing this is by obtaining information from, and joining, a group such as Education Otherwise (see *Useful Contacts*). This national group has supported home education for over 20 years and can give support and practical information, and can inform parents how to deregister the child and what they must do to satisfy the needs of the local education authority. They can also refer parents to specialists within Education Otherwise for special needs and school phobia.

In areas where there are many children being educated at home, there may be local groups of Education Otherwise that meet regularly, so that the children have social interaction with others also not receiving mainstream schooling and parents can talk to other parents and exchange advice.

Conclusion

This chapter has been devoted to severely affected children. Most children affected to this degree will benefit from referral to a specialist child and adolescent mental health service for assessment and therapeutic intervention.

But, regarding the child's education, only the parent can make the final decision on how to best help the child. If parents feel that the child is best served in school, they will reduce the risk of her 'safe' boundaries further diminishing and will also follow current professional thinking on how best to treat a school phobic child. If the school has a special unit that they are prepared to let the child use as a base for her education, this may be a good compromise between full mainstream education and educating the child at home. She will have the security of being involved with fewer children and staff, and may find the atmosphere closer to the one she experiences at home. When she regains her confidence she can be slowly reintegrated into mainstream schooling.

If the only way to keep the child in school is to medicate her (following professional advice), parents may feel it is appropriate to do this or they may feel that regularly forcing the child to attend school, making her physically ill and desperately unhappy for a long period of time, may damage her emotionally.

If parents decide to remove a severely affected child from mainstream schooling, either by educating her themselves or by asking the local education authority to provide tuition, they may view this as either a temporary or permanent option. But whatever decision parents make, it will not be easy. After listening to professional advice, they need to make up their own mind about what is best, as they are the ones who will have to live with the decision and justify it to the child, now or when she is an adult.

If parents choose to take their child out of school, they should remember that they can later change their minds, so it is best not to fall out with the professionals who are involved with the child in case they need to ask them to take her back into school, or to help if things don't go as expected or hoped.

Further reading
Web addresses:

www.aacap.org/publications/factsfam/whenhelp.htm (American Academy of Child and Adolescent Psychiatry webpages on when to get help for the child.)

www.findarticles.com/cf_dls/g2699/0002/2699000201/p1/article.jhtml (Webpage on the learning theory for cognitive behavioural therapy.)

www.beckinstitute.org/training/q&a.htm (The Beck Institute For Cognitive Therapy and Research.)

www.rcpsych.ac.uk/info/factsheets/pfaccog.htm (The Royal College of Psychiatrists' webpages on cognitive therapy.)

members.tripod.com/ernallo/treatmen.htm (This webpage gives a suggested hierarchy of desensitising steps for selective mutism.)

mentalhealth.about.com/library/weekly/aa021698.htm (Wepages on psychotherapy from the Mental Health Resources website.)

www.positivehealth.com/permit/articles/regular/drj.58.htm (Homeopathy for school phobia: written by a homeopathic doctor.)

www.psyc.leeds.ac.uk/research/lftrc/manuals/sft/manual.pdf (A systemic family therapy manual from the Leeds Family Therapy and Research Centre.)

www.motivationalinterview.org/clinical/whatismi.html (A website on motivational interviewing.)

www.smmgp.demon.co.uk/html/articles/art004.htm (A website on motivational interviewing.)

www.getting-on.co.uk/toolkit/brief_extract2.html (Webpages on solution focused brief therapy.)

Books

Milner, J. and O'Byrne, P. (2002) *Brief Counselling: Narratives and Solutions.* New York: Palgrave Macmillian.
Written for practising professionals, this book illustrates how narrative therapy and solution focused brief therapy can be used with clients. Although not written specifically for use with children and adolescents, it does include a chapter that relates to school difficulties.

Graham, P. (ed) (1998) *Cognitive-Behaviour Therapy for Children and Families.* Cambridge: Cambridge University Press.
Written for practising professionals, this book provides a comprehensive account of cognitive behavioural approaches to psychological problems in children, adolescents and their families. Each chapter is written by a different contributor and they progress developmentally, from pre-school to adolescence. Each author focuses on a specific disorder: Chapter Five is devoted to anxiety disorders.

Miller, W.R. and Rollnick, S. (2002) *Motivational Interviewing: Preparing People for Change.* New York: The Guildford Press.
Written for practising professionals, this book has a large body of contributors. Although only one chapter is devoted to using MI with adolescents and young people, the book is extremely thorough in its research and practical applications.

Stallard, P. (2002) *Think Good – Feel Good.* London: John Wiley & Sons.
A workbook to be used with children and young people, covering core elements of CBT. It has a useful introduction to CBT, and photocopiable pages of exercises and worksheets embracing a wide range of psychological problems.

Knox, P. (1988) *Troubled Children: A Fresh Look at School Phobia.* Upton-upon-Severn, UK: Self-published.
This is an extremely well researched book (including many case studies) that compares the education system in Britain with that of other European countries. Ms Knox is also a strong advocate of Education Otherwise, the association of parents who educate their children out of school, and her book is closely linked to the organisation. It offers a very different viewpoint to current professional thinking on the subject and the case studies illustrate some very inhumane professional interventions, which give weight to the argument for home education. Highly recommended for those seriously considering home education for a severely affected child.

Chapter Eight

First Steps in Recovery: Letting Go

When the peak of the child's crisis is over and she starts to show signs of recovery, parents should not be fooled into thinking that they're home and dry. There is still much to be done. They will need to think ahead to predict possible setbacks and weigh up the risks each event has. If they think that there is little chance of the child dealing with something successfully, they should not force her into doing it. They should give her permission to pick and choose what she does.

If she wants to do something but is nervous about it, parents should give the child the support she needs in order to do it, but they should not over-protect her, as she needs to start developing independence again. If she succeeds at something that she wasn't sure about, she will be that bit more confident when a similar situation arises and her feelings of anxiety should be less intense.

Assess how much attention the child needs

When the child is at her most anxious, she will need all the support parents can give her. However, as she gets more confident about things (either to do with school or another part of her life), intensive attention should be withdrawn gradually. Otherwise there is a danger that the child becomes so reliant on her parents that she will eventually want them with her all the time, even when the crisis is over. She may deliberately perpetuate the situation to keep their sympathy.

Once parents think the child can cope with something without their being very attentive (for example, at a party they could hover in the background, rather than have a young child sit on their lap all the way through), they should gently insist that she does it alone. It would be a retrograde step to have the child so in need of her parents that she ceases to function on her own altogether.

Give the child some challenges as soon as she is ready

Parents mustn't give in too easily or rid the child's life of challenges. The challenges should be much smaller than they would have been if there were no problems, but the child should experience a little independence. Once she can cope with this, the goalposts should be moved so that she has to do a bit more.

This is important for two reasons. One is that parents don't want an over-clingy child who needs them for everything: it's too draining on their time and patience – parents need some space and time to themselves. The other reason is that the child needs to relearn independence. If she can gradually discover that there are things she can do alone, without anything bad happening to her, she will regain confidence. And upon each 'layer' of confidence that she regains, another layer can be laid.

One way to identify the suitability of challenges is to discuss with the child all the things she can do now and write them down. Then underneath, make a list of all the things she finds hard or cannot do now (in ascending order of difficulty). If a line were drawn under the things she can do now she could be told that everything above that line she must continue to do without help. Then it could be explained that over the next year or two or three, she is to work slowly down the list. She could have a reward such as a sticker for each step she takes or a special treat. She should be much praised within the family when she can achieve the next step.

Preferably, the child's progress will be made at her own pace, but if too much time elapses between steps she may need encouragement. Parents could give the child a challenge if they think it appropriate. Then the child will need to keep repeating that challenge until she can easily cope with it.

Things to aim for are: attending school with no anxiety at all (first days back after the holidays can be excepted); going to parties alone; being taken out with friends and their main carers; going to after-school clubs; going to sleepovers; staying with relatives without her parents; buying things in shops on her own; answering the 'phone and taking messages; calling friends or relatives to ask a question or relay a message; and going on school trips.

School trips

A school trip is not a regular event. By the time the next one comes, the child's anxieties could be at the same high level even if she went on the first; they are not frequent enough to desensitise her. Parties, however, tend to be much more frequent and trips out can be as often as parents manage to organise them – and they don't have to be expensive, so it is important that the child gradually learns to cope with these.

If the child has not gone anywhere for some time without her parents, going alone with her friends and teachers on a school trip may cause her so much anxiety that she's sick or has a miserable time from constant worrying. This will make her fear the next school trip and so on, enlarging her fears instead of shrinking them. (School trips should be bottom on the child's desensitisation programme: they should only be attempted once the child can easily cope with going out for the day with a friend and her parents.)

If parents feel she cannot cope with a school trip (or really doesn't want to go), the child should not be forced. It is kinder to her and the class teacher, who may find one hysterical child too much to cope with when he or she has the others to mind too (unless her parent is able and willing to go along with her). If the child doesn't go on the trip, being in school without the rest of the class or her teacher may make her very anxious. If this is likely to happen, she should be kept at home until the trip is over (assuming parents are able to do this).

Gradually withdraw support

Just as the child needs to learn to be as independent of her parents as is appropriate to her age, parents have to learn to let go and not over-protect the child because she is anxious. She will stay anxious if she does not learn to do things by herself. When parents think she can cope with the next stage of independence, they should gradually withdraw their support.

When the child is lonely and bored

If parents stop what they are doing every time the child says she's bored she will have no need of friends or of learning to be independent. Constantly amusing the child does not make the perfect parent; that is an impossible and unrealistic state to aspire to. Life has to go on for all members of the family and the child needs to understand this. Parents are not being selfish by refusing to spend time with the child when they are busy. The child can still be in the same room as her parents, while they do whatever they need to.

It should be pointed out to the child that if she does not play with her friends outside school she will lose them, because they all see one another out of school and she's getting left out. If she does this for long, they will lose interest in her. She might say she doesn't care, but it should give her food for thought.

When the child complains of being bored and her parents are genuinely busy, they should explain that they are behind on things because of helping her so much. This should not be said to make her feel guilty, just so that she understands they do not have all day, every day, to devote only to her. Parents can explain that they have needs too and that, right at this moment, theirs are greater than hers. They can tell her that she is welcome to invite a friend round. If she wants her parents to do it for her, they should agree (unless it is felt that this is the 'next stage' and she ought to do it herself).

When the child has been invited to a party

If this is the child's first party since the peak of her anxiety, it is understandable that she will find the idea of going frightening, and will need much support. If the child refuses to leave her parents' side and they feel she should be able to, her parents could tell her that if she doesn't go and play with the other children, they will leave. They could tell her that they did not take her there so she could talk to them; she was taken there for her to be with friends and play (and for her parents to talk to adults). And if she isn't going to do that, they all may as well leave. Parents are there to support her for only as long as they see the child trying to help herself.

If the child can cope with going to a party and is acting independently of her parents while there, the next step is for her to be left at a party on her own. Parents should tell the child that they can't stay with her the whole time but that they'll stay for the first ten minutes and then she must either come back with them (and amuse herself as they have things to do) or stay without them. The child should be told that if she does stay her parents will feel very proud of her. If she doesn't stay, her parents must ensure that what they told her would happen does, but not to make her feel bad about it – just to be neutral.

This approach may seem hard, but for the child's sake parents need to cling on to any independence she has and build upon it. If the child is too anxious to cope with this step right now, parents should ensure that she maintains the level of independence she already has and try another time.

Feeling left out

When friends talk about a film they have been to see together, the child may feel left out and might slowly start thinking in terms of wanting to be in the thick of things and joining friends and their families on outings. However, she may need much help to do this, such as, discussing the exact times she would be out, who would be looking after her, and whether that person understands her problems and knows that she needs to go to the toilet frequently, for example.

Parents can help pave the way for her by taking her and a friend out. She might then accept an invitation out with the friend's family, knowing she felt safe with her friend and that her friend understands. The steps forward should be small and her return to normality unhurried. In this way, progress to independence should be made.

Joining clubs

If possible, the child should be encouraged to join clubs so that she can be occupied and have fun out of school without parental support. Parents may decide the best time to start is in the school holidays, when there is no stress about going to school. Although regular clubs often break up in the holidays, some crash courses in swimming, football or short tennis, for example, may be on offer. These could be checked out at the child's local leisure centre. Stagecoach (details in *Further Resources*), the national theatre school, often does a week's summer course, as do

226 SCHOOL PHOBIA, PANIC ATTACKS AND ANXIETY IN CHILDREN

other organisations. Perhaps the child could do something with a friend?

Dealing with trauma

If something happens to upset the child, such as a bereavement, after she has 'recovered', parents should be prepared for her anxious feelings to return. Separation anxiety can recur in times of stress later in the child's life and parents need to be prepared for this. With older children, they may suffer separation anxiety, for example, when they go to college; it is then called 'homesickness'. With careful handling at the time, any recurrence of symptoms will, hopefully, be quickly resolved.

Remember that how the child responds to a traumatic event depends largely on how her parents respond. Parents should deal with it calmly and matter-of-factly and show the child that life carries on nevertheless, whilst giving sympathy and showing understanding. If the parents are upset too, they should not hide it from the child. She will find it helpful to know that they have feelings too and aren't afraid to express them.

Conclusion

As the child becomes more confident, parents can step further and further into the background. Slow, steady progress is more reassuring at this time to parent and child and they both need to learn what new boundaries the child can achieve, regardless of the knowledge that she used to cope with them. Parents must give the child time and patience and, when she is ready, let go.

Chapter Nine

What to do if the Child Regresses

There is no need to panic if the child regresses. Just because the full measure of the child's anxiety has shown itself before, it doesn't mean it will again, or every time the child becomes anxious. However, parents do need to act quickly and very positively, remembering all the valuable lessons they learned first time round. And they need to be confident in their approach. They are now the expert with the child. No one knows her as well as they and, even if they sought professional help last time, they can probably cope without it this time, and their intervention will be swifter and surer than ever before.

Steps to follow

The steps below should be followed if the child shows signs of panic before school after a long recovery period, if parents are sure that the child has no physical illness (this may be hard to judge, but they can review her recent health to see if she has given signs of becoming more anxious again) and is not being bullied by either another child or her teacher. If an event or series of events is thought to have contributed to the child's dip in confidence, it would be appropriate to follow the steps below:

- Parents should not let any anxiety about the child show in front of the child.

- Parents should not have conversations about the child's condition within her hearing apart from, 'She's fine; just anxious.'

- Parents need to be very firm and tell the child that she still has to go to school, no matter how bad she feels, as it is her anxiety making her feel ill. The only way to beat the anxiety is to carry on as normal and do the same things she usually does.

- The child should be reminded that when she gets involved in school and with her friends, her anxiety will go and so will her feeling ill. It is only through getting involved that she will distract her mind enough to feel better. Parents will not be doing her any favours by letting her stay at home when she does not have a physical illness, because it gets worse – not better – when off school.

- Parents should be understanding; yes the child probably does feel horrible, but because it is not a physical but a mental illness (stemming from negative and anxious thoughts), the only way to deal with it is to do what seems hardest at the time: confront her fears.

- Parents should give the child a positive mantra to use such as, 'I'm fine and will feel better soon. I enjoy being with my friends.'

- Parents should remind the child that she has coped with anxiety before and can again.

- Parents should have the expectation that the child will be fine. Having gone through it before, parents know that giving in compounds the problems. The child has to attend school. They should tell her, 'It seems hard now, but you will be fine.'

- Parents should be deaf to the child's pleadings. They should acknowledge what she says but keep repeating, 'You're not ill even though you feel ill. It is your anxious thoughts that produce the worry hormone in your body that makes you feel ill. The more you worry, the more adrenaline is produced and the more ill you will feel. You can only feel better by distracting your mind and getting involved.'

- Parents should be deaf to the child telling them how horrible they are for making her do something that makes her feel ill. They should say, 'I'm sorry you feel like that. We've been through this before and I've learnt that I'll make things worse for you if I give in. You've got to go to school.'

- Parents should ignore the child's promises and 'deals'. For example, she might say, 'If I can stay at home today, I'll be better for tomorrow. I know I will. I promise I'll go tomorrow, just let me stay at home today.' If parents give in, the chances are it will be even worse tomorrow. If parents have already been down this road, they will know that it's true and this will give them the conviction that they are doing the right thing. A child in panic will agree to anything to avoid the situation, but is unlikely to be able to keep the promise if it is related to attending school.

- Parents should listen to the exact words the child uses. For example, she might say, while on the way to school, 'Just let me come back with you and then I'll be all right. I know I will.' Parents can point out to the child what she has just said. In the example the child knows that she wants to be in the safety of her home. Parents can show the child that she has just told them that it's anxiety that's the problem, that she believes something will happen if she's not at home. They can tell her that it was an unrealistic thought.

- Parents can ring up the school and explain the child is anxious and what they can do to help: 'Could you tell her that she can go to the toilet without asking? And if she's sick, can she have some drink after and some of her lunch? She's not ill so she shouldn't come home: she needs to know that being sick doesn't make any difference – she has to carry on as normal.'

- Parents should praise the child when she gets home for being so brave.

- Parents should ignore the fact that the child tells them she had a rotten day (she may well have done, but giving in to this will give her worse rotten days). She's trying to make her parents feel guilty to achieve her aim: avoidance of the thing that frightens her. Parents could challenge her to tell them of five good things about being in school, if they think it might help.

By being firm and unmoving, explaining that the road of letting the child stay at home has been tried and that it didn't work, parents can gain the child's trust that they have control of the situation, even if she hasn't. The child's problems should quickly resolve in a few weeks.

Match action to the child's age

The child may have been six or seven the last time she had a period of school phobia so it would have been appropriate to tell her friends and ask them for help, or send her off to school with a toy bucket in which to vomit. What was acceptable then may not be so now. As well as worrying about being separated from her parents the child may have become extremely self-conscious.

Does she worry about her friends seeing her parents kiss her goodbye or cuddling her? Is she very concerned about her appearance? Is she starting puberty and is getting spots or blackheads that upset her? Is she concerned about her figure? Or of making a fool of herself in front of others? Does she want her parents to stop being silly in front of her friends or when they are out together?

If this is the case, parents need to modify their behaviour so that the child is not seen to be treated like a young child (such as the kissing and cuddling and silly games) when in public or when her friends are round to play. Parents could try to help reduce her spots and blackheads and listen to her concerns about her clothes and figure. If there is any distorted thinking, they can put it right.

If the child thinks she's going to be sick, parents should let her get on with it without fuss. She can be told afterwards to rinse out her mouth and have a drink. If she thinks she might vomit on the way to school, parents could provide (instead of a toy bucket) a large lunchbox (freezer container or Tupperware box). It has a lid and so the child can safely transport it without it being too obvious if it has something nasty in it. She should be told to empty it and rinse it out when at school and to bring it home to wash.

As the child improves she may not need the lunchbox, but might appreciate a freezer bag (other bags are not strong enough and may leak) so that she does not have to worry about being sick on herself if on a bus or train. The knowledge that there is a ready receptacle may give the child enough confidence not to need it. However, a bag of vomit is harder to manage and will be harder to dispose of than a rigid plastic box. Also, the stomach acid may burn through the plastic and so may only safely hold the vomit for a few minutes.

The child might recover more quickly if her friends aren't told and only a few people know. Even relatives might cause additional problems as they might perceptibly change the way they deal with the child. She is better off with everyone treating her as though there is nothing wrong.

A big advantage when having a recurrence is that the child is probably much older and can now cope with relaxation techniques and cognitive approaches (see Chapter Seven). For example, the child can be asked what the difference is about her school this week. She was fine last week and the months and years before that. So it's obvious that school is not the problem (this should only be said if parents are sure the child is not being bullied and there is no problem with her work). She will then accept that and tell herself that it's not the school she's worried about.

If parents can explain to the child why they think her anxiety has suddenly mounted, it will help. The child should not be fussed over and should be encouraged to do more, not less.

Has the parent unwittingly contributed to what's happened?

Parents should ask themselves if they have contributed to the child's drop in confidence in any way (and admit it to themselves even if not to others) and then take steps to counteract this. For example, if the child has been growing very fast and has had several illnesses close together, she may have felt tired for a long time and have had repeated absences from school. Consequently, her parents may have limited her socialising by saying she was too tired to go out and must rest.

As soon as anxiety kicks in, parents need to reverse such comments and treat the child as completely healthy, letting her go to places and socialise more rather than less (however, if they have genuine concerns, the child can be checked by her doctor first). This does not mean parents should force the child to take up strenuous exercise (if growing fast, her body may not be able to cope). They should just get her out and about with her friends and perhaps take her swimming or go for walks.

Whatever has happened to destroy the child's confidence, parents should try to turn things round using as many ways as they can think of, in as natural and casual a way as possible.

Show the child she is not alone

The film *The Princess Diaries* shows the heroine so terrified of public speaking (at the start of the film) that she runs out of her class to be sick. She is taunted by her classmates but brushes these taunts aside and, later in the film, takes revenge by shoving her ice cream onto another girl's chest. She is clumsy and awkward and her main ambition in life is to be invisible, but she is suddenly pressured into a world of focused attention.

How the girl copes with it and eventually speaks to a grand audience makes interesting and uplifting viewing. Anxious children who watch it will feel she is someone with whom they can empathise. They may also see that the physical posture they adopt has much in common with the heroine's, and can take note that she had to be taught how to stand and walk. Unconfident children often try to reduce the space they take up in an attempt to be less noticeable. But unfortunately, this makes them stand out all the more. At the end of the film the heroine stands tall and confident and seems to enjoy her new role as princess.

The child also shares problems of anxiety with famous people such as:

- John Stuart Mill (1806–1873): British philosopher-economist who had a great impact on 19th-century British thought, not only in philosophy and economics, but also in the areas of political science, logic and ethics.

- Edvard Munch (1863–1944): Norwegian artist who painted *The Scream.*

- Abraham Lincoln (1809–1865): 16th American president.

- Robert Burns (1759–1796): regarded as Scotland's national poet.

- Emily Dickinson (1830–1886): American poet.

- Sir Isaac Newton (1642–1727): British physicist and mathematician.

These people have long departed. A list of contemporary famous people who have suffered from anxiety can be found on the website www.anxietysecrets.com/celebrities.htm. There is also a link to famous people who have been bullied and another for famous people who have had depression and have suffered from other mental health illnesses.

Learn to laugh at the absurdity of some fears

The best way to laugh at some fears is by seeing them for what they are, through the programme *Barking Mad* (details at the end of the chapter), where behaviourists help animal owners solve their pets' problems. (Children should never be taught to laugh at unfortunate people and should not be the butt of jokes themselves.)

To watch a big sturdy horse with water phobia quaking at its approach to a shallow stretch of water before running away in panic is rather funny (for the viewer, but not for the horse or its owner). Other fears horses have had are of carts and jumping (even the lowest of obstacles). Through gradual desensitisation, with the help of a confident behaviourist, all horses recover.

There are dogs, cats and birds with obsessions they are cured of through behaviour therapy, by distracting them when the obsession approaches or is present, and giving them treats to reward them for modifying their behaviour. Other pets are disturbed by their environment, such as not receiving sufficient stimulation and so behaving badly due to boredom, and feeling insecure in their environment, needing a snug and protected place all of their own.

The animals' problems and anxieties are wide ranging and some are brought on by their owners' unwitting behaviour. Each problem shown seems a hard one to tackle, but when the behaviourists explain what they are going to do and why and it is seen to work, the solutions suddenly became obvious – very simple but needing patience and perseverance. The results are amazing.

If the child sees what can be done with these animals and the fears and insecurities they can overcome, she may feel a lot more positive about her own problems and see the need for desensitisation and other techniques. And the parent can take note of the calm and confident manner the behaviourists have when dealing with the animals, to inspire confidence and trust.

Conclusion

Some children may never have school phobia again, but many will. Once a child has shown she has a dependent personality and is very sensitive to new situations, parents will need to be constantly on the watch for their own behaviour and comments, so that they don't put negative ideas into the child's head and so that they quickly redress any loss in the child's confidence before it becomes a big problem. They should note any avoidance behaviour or illness when the child is soon afterwards apparently fine, and take appropriate action. Children such as this need much freedom – not little – and parents may need to work at expanding the child's horizons.

Further reading

Web addresses giving details of famous people with anxiety disorders:

www.algy.com/anxiety/famous.html

www.healthyplace.com/communities/anxiety/paems/people/famous_people_2.htm

www.anxiety-disorders.infoxchange.net.au/famous_people.html

Videos/DVDs

The Best Of Barking Mad (1999) and *The Best Of Barking Mad, Vol. 2* (2002)
These are BBC productions with Phillipa Forrester as presenter. Available from
www.amazon.co.uk, both are suitable for children (and adults) aged five up.

The Princess Diaries (Cert. U)
This film is out on DVD and video. It is suitable for teenagers as well as young
children, particularly girls. It is also ideal for children suffering from social
phobia, as at the start of the film the main character has to talk in front of her
whole class, but is so scared she has to run out to be sick. By the end of the film,
she can speak in front of a large and very important audience.

The Anxious Child

Day is dawning, school this morning
Stomach churning, grips with warning
Filling with dread, won't leave her bed
Frightening thoughts snake through her head
Life is scary, heart pounds wary
Will this fear ever vary?

Take heed my needs, she begs and pleads
She whines and cries 'til she succeeds
Can I not go to school today?
Can I be by your side all day?
I'll calmly play the time away
Promise I won't get in your way

I'll eat my food and I won't brood
I'll be polite and never rude
I won't feel blue or need the loo
Won't be sick or have runny poo
I do not ever wish to sever
My ties with you — no, not ever

The meek and mild anxious child
Feels alone, lost in the wild
Unaware of how she got there
Be kind to her and show some care
Help her fight through this fright
And pass from darkness into light

Give her some hope, help her to cope
But don't shorten the end of her rope
By being her friend right to the end
You'll have a child that for herself can fend
Stay close to her side, be her guide
Then let go for she freely must ride

Further Resources

The following are suggestions of things that could help the child further.

CD

Gloria Gaynor's songs, *I Am What I Am* and *I Will Survive*, found on the compilation CD, *I Will Survive*, have good feisty words to inspire and motivate timid children and young people.

Herbal/complementary remedies

Bach flower remedy: rescue cream

This is intended for use in emergencies including panic and anxiety. It can be rubbed into the child's wrists at her pulse points and on the inside of her elbow. However, suitability and conditions of use should be checked with the pharmacist. The pharmacist may be able to recommend other herbal preparations that could be used to help the child. Although these are unlikely to help a severely affected child, it may be worth giving them a try.

Sea bands

These are inexpensive and available from pharmacists and by mail order. They are elasticised bands worn around the wrists with a hard, raised shape that presses against the child's acupressure point to ease nausea. Some children find these very effective for travel sickness, so they may help a child feeling nauseous before school. However, they do not work for everyone (and didn't with my daughter).

Relaxation/sleep problems
Cassettes and CDs

Ages five to eight: *Keeper of Dreams* (cassette and CD) and *Serenity* (CD): relaxing instrumental music suitable for any age, but I recommend them particularly for this age group as very young children are unable to follow relaxation routines and it can help distract their minds when trying to sleep, without stimulating them as story cassettes can. They are too passive to be used for relaxation for older children, but are still pleasant to listen to.

They are available from: New World Music, The Barn, Becks Green, St Andrews, Beccles, Suffolk NR34 8NB, England. Tel: 01986 781682. Website: www.newworldmusic.com.

DR NIAL REYNOLDS' CASSETTES

Ages eight to adult: *Grey Squirrel* relaxation cassettes: although these were made for adults, they are the only recordings I know of that are also suitable for this age group. Each cassette has two sessions lasting about half an hour and, after a brief relaxation routine, a soothing, magical story is told in Dr Reynolds' grandfatherly voice. The recordings can be used purely for relaxation at any time of the day as there is a wake-up sequence at the end – or they can be used at bedtime and can be switched off before the wake-up sequence starts.

The repetitiveness of having the same story/stories told each night may make the *Grey Squirrel* recordings suitable for children with Asperger syndrome. And because the relaxation routine at the start is so brief (and without the need to learn diaphragmatic breathing), there is little pressure to try to maintain a relaxed state; consequently, this is less likely to make a child with Asperger syndrome more anxious. (This section could be skipped for such a child if it proved to be anxiety-provoking.) However, for other children, it can help them relax as it involves tensing and relaxing muscle groups.

- *Relax with Grey Squirrel 1*: Listeners are introduced to Grey Squirrel in the first session and, in the second, listeners hear the story of his Christmas party.

- *Relax with Grey Squirrel 2*: Listeners are told *The Story of the Copper Beech Tree* and *The Island in the Reservoir*.

- *Relax with Grey Squirrel 3*: Listeners are told the story of *How Grey Squirrel got a Bushy Tail* and *The Story of the Pumpkin Seeds*.

It is extremely useful having a gentle story to listen to when in a relaxed state as it distracts the mind from worrying thoughts and maintains, even deepens, the child's state of relaxation, allowing her to drift off to sleep (if used as a sleep aid).

Ages ten to adult: *Deep Sleep* cassette: although this recording was made for adults, older children can also use it; the vocabulary is more difficult than in the *Grey Squirrel* recordings. There are six sessions, each beginning with brief relaxation that focuses on breathing and muscle tension, then a visualisation of journeys through, for example, beautiful countryside, a waterfall and a rainbow. Each session lasts 12–15 minutes.

Prior to printing this book, Dr Nial Reynolds passed over the distribution of these recordings to me, following my interest in including them in this book, as he plans to retire. They are available from: Márianna Csóti, c/o St Donat's Castle, Llantwit Major, Vale of Glamorgan CF61 1WF. (£8 each inc. p&p in the UK, payable by cheque, made out to Márianna Csóti.) For postal enquiries, please include a SAE; for enquiries by email, write to: marianna.csoti@ virgin.net. My website is: www.bookstohelppeople.co.uk. Prices are guaranteed until at least September 2004.

I had a library of sleep/relaxation cassettes for the students in my care (in my role as houseparent) and I lent these out when the students were stressed, had anxiety problems or had trouble sleeping. I also loaned personal cassette players and fast battery chargers with four rechargeable batteries so that the students were supplied with a complete package. Residential care workers might consider doing this for those in their care.

Once the earlier cassettes have been mastered, children can move on to adult half-hour relaxation cassettes that do not necessarily involve stories and visualisation. A selection can be obtained from: The Inner Bookshop, 111 Magdalen Road, Oxford OX4 1RQ. Tel: 01856 245 301. Or visit their website at www.innerbookshop.com.

Some relaxation cassettes are reviewed on www.relaxation.clara.net, but none are specifically for children.

Theatre schools

Stagecoach theatre school is a worldwide organisation that has local groups through franchises; it is, however, expensive. But the children get professional tuition in dancing, singing and drama and there is a limit of 15 children per class. There are several classes with different age groups. Both boys and girls attend and teachers are of both sexes; the dancing is modern so boys need not fear a 'ballet' approach. Stagecoach also runs week-long summer courses. Look in your local paper to see if there is a school in your area or investigate the website at www.stage-coach.co.uk/indexhighest.htm.

Italia Conti Associate Schools are part-time theatre schools, mainly in the south-east of the UK. To find out if there's a school in your area ring Sam Newton on 01483 568070.

Sylvia Young Theatre School has Saturday and holiday (residential) schools in London (near Baker St and Marylebone stations) for all age groups. To find out more, go to home.freeuk.com/sylviayoung or ring 020 7402 0673.

Useful Contacts

Bullying

Anti-Bullying Campaign
185 Tower Bridge Road
London SE1 2UF
020 7378 1446
Provides help for bullied children and for children who bully

Bullying Online
www.bullying.co.uk

Childwatch
19 Spring Bank
Hull
East Yorkshire HU3 1AF
01482 325 552
For confidential help and advice or just a chat
www.childwatch.org.uk
Gives advice on bullying and abuse that occur at home and at school for children and adults

Childline
Studd Street
London N1 0QW
020 7239 1000
0800 1111
24-hour helpline for children
www.childline.org.uk
Telephone service for all children and young people, providing confidential counselling, support and advice on any issue. Children can also write to Childline, who answer all letters

Commission for Racial Equality
St Dunstan's House
201–211 Borough High Street
London SE1 1GZ
020 7939 0000
www.cre.gov.uk
Organisation working against racism

Kidscape
2 Grosvenor Gardens
London SW1W 0DH
020 7730 3300
www.kidscape.org.uk/kidscape
Charity set up to protect children from danger – whether from peers, adults they know or strangers

Institute of Race Relations
2–6 Leeke Street
King's Cross Road
London WC1X 9HS
020 7837 0041/020 7833 2010
www.irr.org.uk
This organisation is 'at the cutting edge of research and analysis that informs the struggle for racial justice in Britain and internationally'

NSPCC (National Society for the Prevention of Cruelty to Children)
Weston House
42 Curtain Road
London EC2A 3NH
020 7825 2500
Helpline: 0808 800 5000
www.nspcc.org.uk

Parentline
Endway House
Endway
Hadleigh
Essex SS7 2AN
01702 554782
Helpline: 0808 800 2222
ds.dial.pipex.com/town/plaza/gfm15
Telephone helpline for parents under stress. It offers help and advice on bringing up children and teenagers

National Association of Victim Support Schemes
Cranmer House
39 Brixton Road
London SW9 6DZ
020 7735 9166
natiasso03.uuhost.uk.uu.net
Charity to help victims of crime

Eating Disorders

Eating Disorders Association
103 Prince of Wales Road
Norwich NR1 1DW
Adult helpline: 0845 634 1414 Youthline: 0845 634 7650 www.edauk.com
Information and support for sufferers of anorexia, bulimia and other eating disorders, and their families

Education

Advisory Centre for Education (ACE)
1c Aberdeen Studios
22 Highbury Grove
London N5 2DQ
020 7704 9822 (exclusion line)
0808 800 5793 (general advice Mon–Fri, 2–5pm)
www.ace-ed.org.uk
Information and advice on any aspect of state education. Helps parents or carers when dealing with schools and education authorities

Education Otherwise
PO Box 7420
London N9 9SG
0870 730 0074 (recorded details of contacts) www.education-otherwise.org
*Support, advice and information to families practising or contemplating home-based
education as an alternative to school*

School House Home Education Association
311 Perth Road
Dundee DD2 1LG
0870 745 0968
0870 745 0967
24-hour information line
www.schoolhouse.org.uk
*Information and support for parents throughout Scotland interested in home-based
education*

Include
www.include.org.uk
*National charity dedicated to tackling the crisis of social exclusion among young people.
National projects helping children and young people aged 5–19 back into education,
training or employment who have not attended for a variety of reasons, including school
exclusion*

Health

Action for ME
PO Box 1302
Wells
Somerset BA5 1YE
01749 670799
www.actionforme.org.uk
Information and support for sufferers of CFS/ME

The ME Association
4 Top Angel
Buckingham Industrial Park
Buckingham MK18 1TH
01280 818964 Information line: 01280 816115
www.meassociation.org.uk
Information and support for sufferers of CFS/ME

Mental Health and Counselling

Anxiety Care
Cardinal Heenan Centre
326 High Road
Ilford
Essex IG1 1QP
020 8262 8891/2 Helpline: 020 8478 3400
www.anxietycare.org.uk
Helps sufferers of anxiety-related problems

British Association for Counselling and Psychotherapy
1 Regent Place
Rugby
Warks CV21 2PJ
0870 443 5252
www.bac.co.uk
Lists counsellors all over the UK, and gives information and advice

The British Psychological Society
St Andrew's House
48 Princess Road East
Leicester LE1 7DR
0116 254 9568
www.bps.org.uk/index.cfm
If parents want to consult a psychologist privately, they can supply a list of those in their area

Childline
As above

Cruse Bereavement Care
Cruse House
126 Sheen Road
Richmond
Surrey TW9 1UR
Helpline: 0870 167 1677 Counselling line: 08457 585565
home.freeuk.net/cruselochaber/canhelp.html
Offers help and counselling to anyone who has suffered bereavement

ERIC (Enuresis Resource and Information Centre)
34 Old School House
Britannia Road
Kingswood
Bristol BS15 8DB
0117 960 3060
www.eric.org.uk
Offers information and advice about day and night wetting to parents, young people and professionals

National Phobics Society
Zion Community Resource Centre
339 Stretford Road
Hulme
Manchester M15 4ZY
0870 7700 456
www.phobics-society.org.uk
Information and support for phobias, anxiety, panic attacks and compulsive disorders

Obsessive Action
Aberdeen Centre
22–24 Highbury Grove
London N5 2EA
020 7226 4000
www.obsessive-action.demon.co.uk
National organisation for people with obsessive compulsive disorder

Royal College of Psychiatrists
17 Belgrave Square
London SW1X 8PG
020 7235 2351
www.rcpsych.ac.uk
Factsheets on Mental Health and Growing Up *available*

SANE
1st Floor
Cityside House
40 Adler Street
London E1 1EE
020 7375 1002 Saneline: 0845 767 8000
www.sane.org.uk
Helping people cope with mental illness

Samaritans
The Upper Mill
Kingston Road
Ewelly
Surrey KT17 2AF
020 8394 8300 National helpline: 08457 909090 www.samaritans.org.uk
24-hour help to people who feel suicidal or desperate for any reason

YoungMinds
102–108 Clerkenwell Road
London EC1M 5SA
020 7336 8445
Parent's information service: 0800 018 2138
www.youngminds.org.uk
For parents or carers with concerns about the mental health or emotional well being of a child or young person

Special Educational Needs

British Dyslexia Association
98 London Road
Reading RG1 5AU
0118 966 2677 Helpline: 0118 966 8271
www.bda-dyslexia.org.uk

Contact a Family
209–211 City Road
London EC1V 1JN
020 7608 8700 Helpline: 0808 808 3555
www.cafamily.org.uk
Support and advice for families with disabled children or those suffering from any medical condition

IPSEA (Independent Panel for Special Education Advice)
6 Carlow Mews
Woodbridge
Suffolk IP12 1EA
01394 380518 Advice line: 0800 018 4016
www.ipsea.org.uk
Gives information and advice concerning special educational needs

National Association for Special Educational Needs (NASEN)
NASEN House
4–5 Amber Business Village
Amber Close
Amington
Tamworth B77 4RP
01827 311500
www.nasen.org.uk/mainpg.htm
Support for parents or carers and professionals who are concerned with special educational needs

The National Autistic Society
393 City Road
London EC1V 1NG
020 7833 2299
www.nas.org.uk
For children and adults with autism and Asperger syndrome

Mencap National Centre
123 Golden Lane
London EC1Y 0RT
020 7454 0454
www.mencap.org.uk
Services, advice and support for people with learning difficulties, their families and their carers

Subject Index

Name Index